# Edge-to-Edge Mitral Repair

Ottavio Alfieri • Michele De Bonis
Giovanni La Canna
Editors

# Edge-to-Edge Mitral Repair

From a Surgical to a Percutaneous
Approach

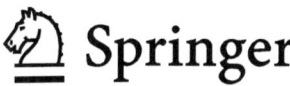 Springer

*Editors*
Ottavio Alfieri
Department of Cardiac Surgery
San Raffaele Hospital
Milan
Italy

Giovanni La Canna
Department of Cardiac Surgery
San Raffaele Hospital
Milan
Italy

Michele De Bonis
Department of Cardiac Surgery
San Raffaele Hospital
Milan
Italy

ISBN 978-3-319-19892-7       ISBN 978-3-319-19893-4    (eBook)
DOI 10.1007/978-3-319-19893-4

Library of Congress Control Number: 2015946864

Springer Cham Heidelberg New York Dordrecht London

Printed on acid-free paper

Springer International Publishing AG Switzerland is part of Springer Science+Business Media
(www.springer.com)

This book on edge-to-edge mitral valve repair represents a remarkable compendium because it is organized and edited by the inventor of the technique and incorporates a perspective that has been shaped by two decades of development. This path of development has been controversial, sparking debates about the optimal methods for surgical repair for mitral regurgitation (MR) and serving as the basis for the beginning of the new field of percutaneous therapy for MR. All of these issues are contained and addressed within this text, which is unique for its depth on this subject.

The surgical edge-to-edge technique gave rise to percutaneous edge-to-edge with the MitraClip. Remarkably, the visibility of percutaneous repair has raised awareness of the utility of surgical edge-to-edge among the surgical community. I have been interested to see many surgeons, who were often highly critical of the edge-to-edge repair, come to adopt the use of surgical edge-to-edge when conventional annuloplasty is insufficient, with recognition that edge-to-edge can be a predictor of better surgical outcomes than isolated annuloplasty. A greater understanding of edge-to-edge has led to lessened concerns and some of the early doubts about the technique, such as distortion of the leaflets or the creation of mitral stenosis as complications.

Several important questions about the physiology of edge-to-edge are not widely understood. The mechanism by which the annulus appears to stabilize by isolated edge-to-edge is speculative. The distribution of forces on the mitral leaflets after edge-to-edge has been modeled, but it still seems surprising that these forces do not result in early failure of the sutures that are used for this technique. This book will help the reader understand how it is possible for the technique to have early success. The congenital double orifice mitral valve served as the inspiration for this surgical approach, and its existence as a bystander finding rather than a clinical problem is a model for recognizing that the surgical double orifice is tolerated by patients.

The chapter on echocardiography reflects the growing importance of imaging in surgery for MR. The role of imaging has become increasingly integrated into both assessment and intra-procedural guidance. We can only go where we can see, and the greater understanding that has come from three-dimensional echo for MR diagnosis and procedural decision making is part of today's practice.

Perhaps the greatest contribution of the edge-to-edge concept has been the dialog and interchange that it has stimulated among surgeons, interventional cardiologists, and recently heart failure specialists. In his seminal 1998 paper on this technique in the *European Journal of Cardiothoracic Surgery*, Professor Alfieri wrote,

"Eventually, the concept introduced by this type of repair can open the perspective of percutaneous correction of MR." This statement has been prescient. It was the stimulus for the development of the MitraClip and other catheter-based attempts to mimic the edge-to-edge repair. These efforts led at first to controversy, which then became debate and is now part of the daily heart team dialog that has become an integral part of decision making and treatment for valvular heart disease. This dialog occurs in most heart valve "centers of excellence" and is part of all of our conferences on valve therapy.

Professor Alfieri and I met at the first meeting on percutaneous valve therapy in London in April 2004. The meeting was unique because it brought together surgeons and interventional cardiologists with an interest in valve therapy. I clearly remember the mutual interest we shared in developing better methods for treating MR, with the recognition that everyone involved had something to contribute to the effort. This book represents the continuation of that journey and spirit with contributions from specialists from different disciplines and representing over two decades of experience and growing knowledge about treating MR generally and specifically about edge-to-edge repair.

Ted Feldman, MD, FESC, FACC, MSCAI
NorthShore University Health System
Evanston, IL, USA

# Contents

# The Genesis of the Edge-to-Edge Technique

Ottavio Alfieri

Not surprisingly, in surgery new solutions are explored and new methods are developed when the available techniques are not entirely satisfactory and results are suboptimal. A strong motivation to look for alternative options can also be determined by the complexity of the currently used procedures, particularly demanding, time consuming, and difficult to reproduce.

To put the genesis of the edge-to-edge technique in the right perspective, the scenario of mitral valve repair in the early 1990s has to be taken into account.

## 1.1 The Scenario of Mitral Valve Repair in the Early 1990s

Already at that time, mitral valve repair, popularized by Carpentier et al. [1] was carried out in several institutions around the world, and it was considered by many surgeons the preferred method to treat patients with degenerative mitral regurgitataion.

The superiority of valve repair over valve replacement was clearly established.

Advantages associated with mitral repair were well summarized by Perrier et al. [2]: better preservation of left ventricular function, avoidance of prosthetic related events, reduced hospital mortality and morbidity, shorter postoperative hospital stay, improved long-term survival.

The surgical principles to obtain a good surface of leaflets coaptation and therefore a long-lasting mitral valve repair were also already well defined and the outcome of the procedures was generally predictable.

O. Alfieri, MD, PhD
Cardiac Surgery Unit, IRCCS San Raffaele University Hospital,
Via Olgettina 60, Milan 20132, Italy
e-mail: alfieri.ottavio@hsr.it

© Springer International Publishing Switzerland 2015
O. Alfieri et al. (eds.), *Edge-to-Edge Mitral Repair: From a Surgical to a Percutaneous Approach*, DOI 10.1007/978-3-319-19893-4_1

However, at that time the overall repair rate in the surgical community was still rather low, mainly due to the complexity and/or uneffectiveness of some peculiar techniques.

Moreover, the results of mitral repair in some subsets of lesions appeared to be definitely suboptimal even in experienced hands. For instance, hemodynamically significant residual or recurrent mitral regurgitation was not uncommon after correction of anterior mitral prolapse/flail, bileaflet prolapse, and commissural prolapse, as repeatedly reported in several studies [3–6].

On the contrary, the prolapse of the posterior leaflet, by far the most common lesion in degenerative mitral regurgitation, was associated with satisfactory short and long-term results [3].

Considering all the above, it was quite clear that in the early 1990s there was some space for improvement in mitral valve repair.

In 1990, Frater et al. reported the initial clinical experience with chordal replacement using ePTFE material in 14 patients [7]. Although encouraging results were obtained in that small series, the great potential of chordal replacement was not immediately appreciated and for a while this technique was not widely applied to correct prolapse / flail in mitral valve repair.

The appropriate length of the artificial chordae to be implanted appeared to be a difficult technical issue, and, in addition, long-term results were not available.

In my view, a simple and effective technique to correct some subsets of mitral lesions was badly needed at that time.

## 1.2    The First Case

The first edge-to-edge mitral valve repair was inspired by the observation of a rare congenital anomaly, the double-orifice mitral valve, in a young patient who underwent surgical correction of a large atrial septal defect. In that patient, the mitral valve which was carefully inspected through the atrial septal defect, was perfectly competent. This observation gave me the idea of reproducing surgically the double-orifice configuration to correct mitral regurgitation in selected patients. Therefore, in a patient with severe mitral regurgitation due to the prolapse of the central segment of the anterior leaflet, who was operated by me later on the same day (April 25 1991), the prolapsing portion of the anterior leaflet was sutured to the facing part of the posterior leaflet, and a double-orifice competent valve was obtained. The operation was completed with the insertion of a prosthetic ring, to improve leaflet coaptation and to stabilize the reconstruction, according to the standard practice in the surgical repair of degenerative mitral disease.

Due to the large native mitral annulus, no mitral stenosis was created.

After this first successfully performed edge-to-edge repair, I immediately had the perception that such a procedure could have an impact of some relevance in the treatment of patients with mitral regurgitation.

As a matter of fact, the functional result was perfect: the newly created double-orifice mitral valve was totally competent, and the global mitral valve area was well above 3 cm$^2$, even after implantation of a prosthetic ring.

Besides being effective, the edge-to-edge repair was extraordinarily simple.

Only few minutes were required to correct a lesion which was considered complex and well known to be historically associated with unsatisfactory surgical results. At that time many surgeons used to replace the native mitral valve with a prosthesis, when the anterior leaflet prolapse/flail was identified as the mechanism producing mitral regurgitation.

It was clear to me after this initial case that a double-orifice repair could be easily reproducible by every surgeon and therefore be a useful addition to the armamentarium of the techniques used for mitral valve reconstructive surgery.

## 1.3   Initial Experience, Refinements and Validation

Initially, the edge-to-edge technique was applied with caution, exclusively in those cases where unsatisfactory results could have been anticipated using conventional methods of mitral repair, or when the mechanism of mitral regurgitation was not clear.

Only the most challenging and demanding situations therefore were treated with the new procedure.

Indeed, the edge-to-edge repair was never applied for segmental posterior leaflet prolapse or flail, a lesion which was known to be associated with excellent short and long-term results using a well established and effective technique, the quadrangular resection.

The decision to proceed with caution and to apply the new technique only in a limited and well selected patient population was due to the awareness that sufficiently long follow-up data were not available.

Furthermore, the great enthusiasm for the procedure was somehow mitigated by the skepticism of the surgical community. The main criticism was that the edge-to-edge repair was not reproducing the configuration of a normal mitral valve and was a sort of convenient short cut for those who were unable to properly reconstruct the mitral valve. The occurrence of mitral stenosis was considered a potential problem, and the long-term durability of a double-orifice mitral valve was questioned.

Technical refinements and adjustments were gradually introduced over time, and the technique was standardized, with the adoption of some modifications according to the anatomical features of the individual valve.

Some rules have to be respected in order to apply the procedure correctly.

First of all, the suture connecting the leaflets should be corresponding to the zone of the regurgitant jet. When the regurgitant jet is located in the central part of the mitral valve, the suture produces a mitral valve with a double-orifice configuration (double-orifice repair) (Fig. 1.1). Depending on the precise location of the suture performed along the line of coaptation, the two orifices can have similar or different sizes.

When the jet of regurgitation is in the proximity of a commissure, the edge-to-edge suture results in a mitral valve with a single orifice, smaller in size than the original one (paracommissural repair) (Fig. 1.2).

**Fig. 1.1** Double-orifice
edge-to-edge repair

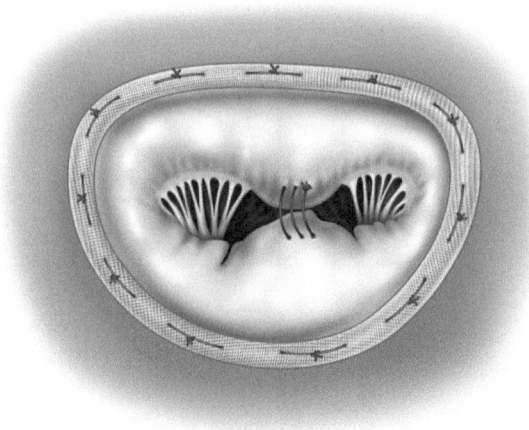

**Fig. 1.2** Paracommissural
edge-to-edge repair

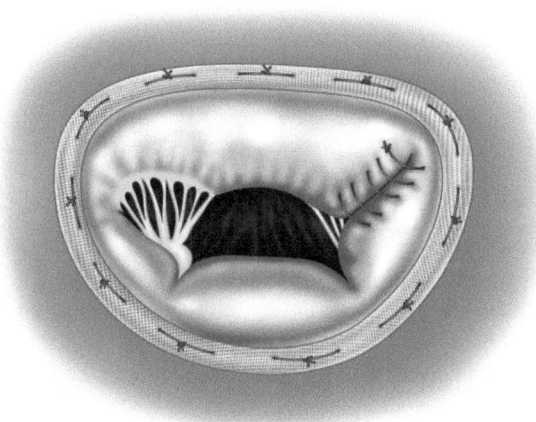

The suture connecting the leaflets should respect the symmetry of the valve and not create any distortion.

The extension of the suture should be as limited as possible: enough to correct mitral regurgitation without producing mitral stenosis. The competence of the valve is evaluated intraoperatively by forceful injection of saline solution into the left ventricle, while the global valve area is assessed by introducing Hegar dilators into the valve orifices.

The distance of the suture bites from the free edges of the leaflets should be variable, according to the redundancy of the valve tissue. The more redundancy is present, the more distant from the free edge the stitches should be, in order to reduce the height of the leaflet and minimize the likelihood of postoperative systolic anterior motion (SAM).

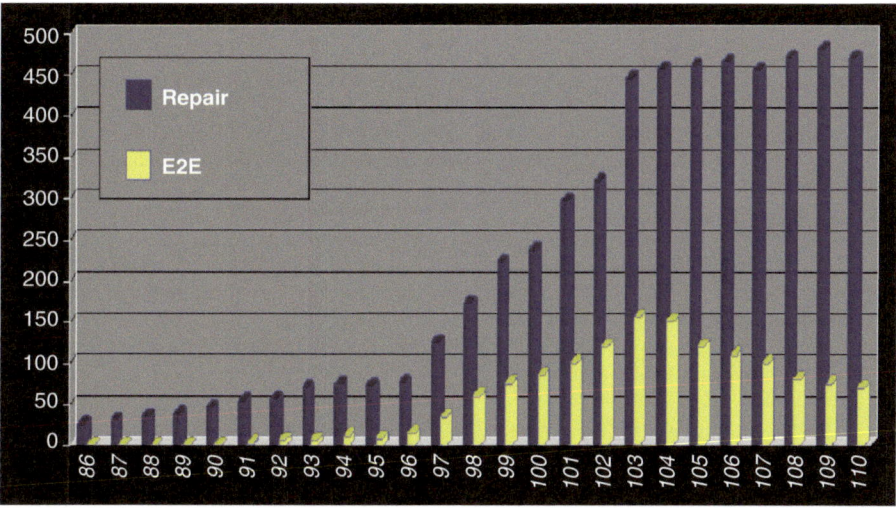

**Fig. 1.3** Rate of adoption of the edge-to-edge technique at San Raffaele University Hospital over the years (*blue columns*: overall number of isolated mitral valve repair procedures per year; *yellow columns*: edge-to-edge repairs per year)

The edge-to-edge suture is conveniently reinforced with teflon pledgets only when the leaflets are very thin, almost transparent as occasionally seen in case of fibro-elastic deficiency.

According to the general principles of mitral valve reconstructive surgery, a prosthetic ring annuloplasty is considered an important step of the operation and is routinely added to the repair at the level of the leaflets.

When the above listed technical aspects are taken into account, the edge-to-edge repair is invariably successful in restoring a well functioning mitral valve.

The appropriate technique has been developed gradually over time and therefore the genesis of the edge-to-edge procedure has been an ongoing process for a while.

From the genesis to the present time, the worldwide experience with the edge-to-edge technique expanded, and the validity of the concept was repeatedly demonstrated in a variety of subsets and clinical scenarios.

Rigorous follow-up data were collected including echo findings at rest and under exercise, and highly satisfactory long-term results (up to 20 years) were reported.

In addition, the pathophysiology of the operation was extensively studied using computer modeling methods.

The most convincing proof of the validity of the edge-to-edge technique as a method to correct complex mitral regurgitation is the extraordinary increase in referral for mitral valve repair at the S. Raffaele University Hospital. As shown in Fig. 1.3, the number of patients submitted to mitral valve repair in our institution was constantly and consistently increasing over the years, with a rate of adoption of the edge-to-edge technique ranging from 15 to 35 %.

# References

1. Carpentier A. Cardiac valve surgery – the "french correction". J Thorac Cardiovasc Surg. 1983;86:323–37.
2. Perier P, Deloche A, Chauvaud S, et al. Comparative evaluation of mitral valve repair and replacement with Starr, Bjork, and porcine valves bioprostheses. Circulation. 1984;70: 187–92.
3. Baunberger E, Deloche A, Berrebi A, et al. Very long-term results ( more than 20 years) of valve repair with Carpentier's technique in non-rheumatic mitral valve insufficiency. Circulation. 2001;104:I8–11.
4. Mohty D, Orszulak TA, Schaff HV, et al. Very long-term survival and durability of mitral valve repair for mitral valve prolapse. Circulation. 2001;104:I1–7.
5. Gillinov AM, Consgrove DM, Blackstone EH, et al. Durability of mitral valve repair for degenerative disease. J Thorac Cardiovasc Surg. 1998;111:734–43.
6. David TE, Ivanov J, Armstrong S, et al. A comparison of outcomes of mitral valve repair for degenerative disease with posterior, anterior or bileaflet prolapse. J Thorac Cardiovasc Surg. 2005;130:1242–9.
7. Frater RW, Vetter HO, Zussa C, et al. Chordal replacement in mitral valve repair. Circulation. 1990;82:152–8.

# The Principle: From a Computational Model to Clinical Validation

Francesco Sturla, Emiliano Votta, Maurizio Taramasso, Andrea Guidotti, Alberto Redaelli, and Francesco Maisano

In the early phase of the clinical experience with the Alfieri technique, we were confronted with several unanswered questions in search for an urgent answer. While the technique seemed to be reliable and easy to apply in different settings, the clinical and pathophysiological consequences of creating a double-orifice valve were unknown. The main questions were concerning the hemodynamics of a double-orifice valve: How much the double-orifice configuration affects diastolic transmitral flow? How is the transmitral flow after a symmetric vs. asymmetric double-orifice repair? Are Doppler derived hemodynamics a reliable method to assess transmitral flow dynamics? What is the risk of leaflet tear? What is the risk of generating mitral stenosis when a ring is added to the Alfieri technique? Is turbulent flow associated with higher risk of thromboembolism?

The acute effects of the therapy were impressive. The simplicity, versatility, and reproducibility of the edge-to-edge (EE) procedure became soon evident, but the above-mentioned questions raised several doubts regarding the safety and the durability of it.

The conventional method to determine the effects of a novel therapy would have implied the design of a clinical study, collecting clinical as well as imaging data to analyze the clinical outcomes and address the pathophysiological issues related to the "non-physiologic" creation of a valve with two orifices. However, such an approach would have required long follow-up time and large numbers to provide reasonable and clinically meaningful answers. In search for a faster solution to obtain these stringent clinical questions, computer modeling was adopted. Most questions raised by the new technique were merely based on the structural and hemodynamic consequences of the suture between the leaflets, a condition that

F. Sturla • E. Votta • A. Redaelli
Department of Electronics, Information and Bioengineering, Politecnico di Milano, Italy

M. Taramasso • A. Guidotti • F. Maisano (✉)
Division of Cardiovascular Surgery, University Hospital of Zurich, Zurich, Switzerland
e-mail: francesco.maisano@usz.ch

© Springer International Publishing Switzerland 2015
O. Alfieri et al. (eds.), *Edge-to-Edge Mitral Repair: From a Surgical to a Percutaneous Approach*, DOI 10.1007/978-3-319-19893-4_2

would easily fit in a computer modeling assessment. Computer models can be effectively used to study the general behavior of a simulated procedure and guide more focused clinical trials. As a result, computational analysis has been successfully applied in cardiovascular research to investigate on surgical and diagnostic procedures and is a valuable alternative to in vitro studies [1, 2].

The increasing sophistication of surgical solutions and the broad range of potential percutaneous strategies necessitate the development of quantitative patient-specific numerical tools, thus requiring an effective integration between state-of-the-art clinical imaging and current finite element approaches. For this purpose, more refined and realistic modeling approaches have been progressively developed exploiting in vivo biomedical imaging techniques to achieve a patient-specific description of MV anatomy and associated dysfunctions.

Computational studies, although limited by the simplification of the models, have the advantage of abolishing the inter-individual variability of clinical and anatomical presentation, and allow investigation of single topics, independent from the surrounding conditions and the large number of confounders that may influence clinical outcomes.

## 2.1    Effects on MV Orifice Dynamics and Hemodynamics

The presence of the edge-to-edge deeply modifies the configuration of the leaflets; based on the tight interrelation between MV substructures, possible indirect effects on the annulus and on the subvalvular apparatus have been speculated. Moreover, the reduction of the area available for diastolic transmitral flow has raised questions regarding the risk of stenosis.

In order to answer the abovementioned unsolved arising questions, computational model of a double-orifice mitral valve based on the finite elements method was used to assess the hemodynamic effects of the repair [3, 4]. In particular, this model was developed to address three of the main issues arising from clinical experience:

1. Is the hemodynamic performance of the mitral valve affected by the configuration of the orifice (single vs. double orifice)?
2. Does the design of the double-orifice valve influence the hemodynamics (orifices of equal vs. unequal areas)?
3. How Doppler-derived flow velocity analysis should be used to determine pressure gradients through the valve under the conditions of a double-orifice flow pattern?

Nine different geometries were investigated, corresponding to three total inflow areas (1.5, 2.25, and 3 cm$^2$) and to three orifice configurations (two equal orifices, two orifices of different areas, i.e., one twice as much as the other one, and a single orifice) (Fig. 2.1). All the geometrical configurations were tested under different flow regimens.

**Fig. 2.1** (**a**)
3D-reconstruction of the left
heart, (**d**) meshed cross-
section of the mitral valve
with a single-orifice
configuration, (**b**) meshed
cross-section of the mitral
valve with a double-orifice
configuration, (**c**) meshed
cross-section of the mitral
valve with double-orifice
configuration (two orifices of
different areas)

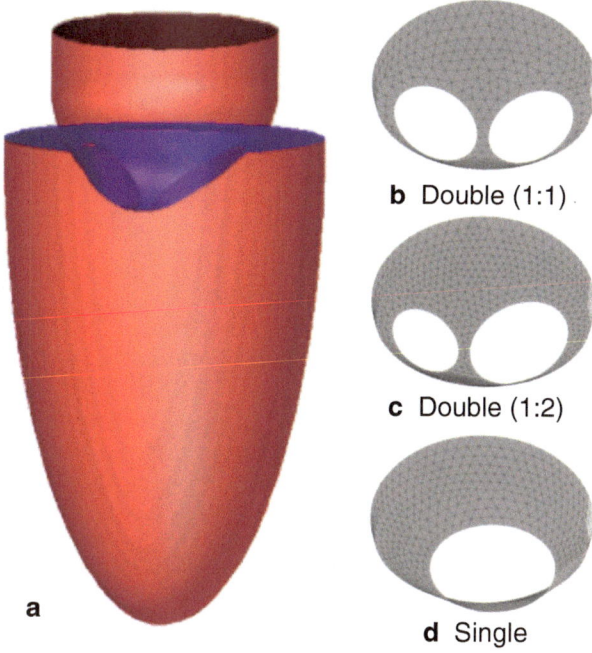

**b** Double (1:1)

**c** Double (1:2)

**a**

**d** Single

The simulation of the fluid dynamics through single- and double-orifice mitral valves showed that the velocity of the blood – and hence the pressure gradients – is exclusively influenced by the total valve area (either as a single area or the sum of two areas) and it does not depend on the conformation of the orifices. In double-orifice valve configuration, the velocity of the flow through each orifice is very similar to the one observed through a single-orifice valve of area equal to the sum of the areas of the two orifices (Fig. 2.2a, b)

Moreover, the velocities of the blood through the two orifices are very similar regardless of the ratio between the areas of the two orifices (Fig. 2.2b, c). This finding warrants the applicability of echo-Doppler examination for the assessment of the results of valve repair by means of non-invasive methods. During echo-Doppler examination, the flow through the valve can be probed at any of the two orifices, obtaining data on overall valve performance (flow velocity, pressure gradient, functional valve area).

The results of the simulation gave to the clinical community fundamental answers which contributed to the progressive diffusion and adoption of the edge-to-edge technique.

Subsequently, initial clinical experience with the Alfieri repair confirmed these findings: In a preliminary series of ten patients, previously submitted to double-orifice repair, in sinus rhythm, the velocities recorded at each orifice by Doppler examination did not differ by more than 5 % [3]. According to the simulation results, the maximum velocity was recorded laterally with respect to the center of the orifice. Simulations show that the lateral velocity can be considerably higher than the

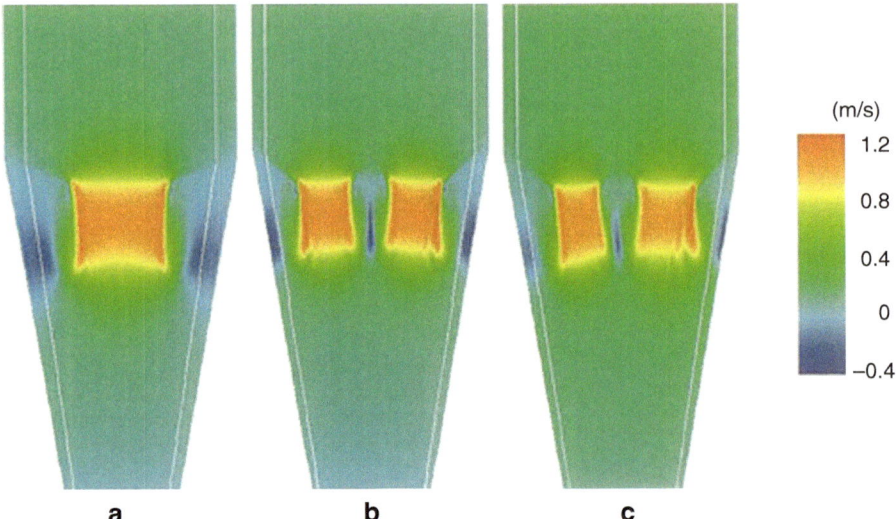

**Fig. 2.2** Velocity colour map for simulations (**a**) single orifice, (**b**) double orifice with equal, and (**c**) unequal areas (Reproduced with permission from [3])

central one. Consequently, the underestimation of the pressure gradients was notably, up to 35 %, when the maximum velocity at the center of the jets was considered for the pressure drop calculations.

The simulation showed that the pattern of pressure fields within the ventricle during diastolic flow is similar either with a single-orifice or a double-orifice valve (Fig. 2.3). The only variation is in the subvalvar area, while the pattern in the atrium and in the middle zone and at the apex of the ventricle does not change. Moreover, the model showed an important pressure recovery within the ventricle (about 20 %), downstream of the valvular plane, thus indicating that the kinetic energy of the jet is not completely dissipated. This was not influenced either by the configuration (single vs. double orifice) or by the shape (equal or different orifices) of the valve.

Summarizing, the model gave precise answers to the abovementioned questions, demonstrating that:

1. The hemodynamic performance of a double-orifice mitral valve is the same of that of a single-orifice valve with an effective orifice area equivalent to the sum of the two orifices.
2. The ratio between the orifice areas does not influence the hemodynamics of the valve.
3. Doppler-derived velocities are a good indicator of hemodynamics and, more specifically, of pressure loss through the valve.

These findings supported the reliability of the double-orifice repair for the treatment of mitral regurgitation, and allowed estimation of the results by noninvasive

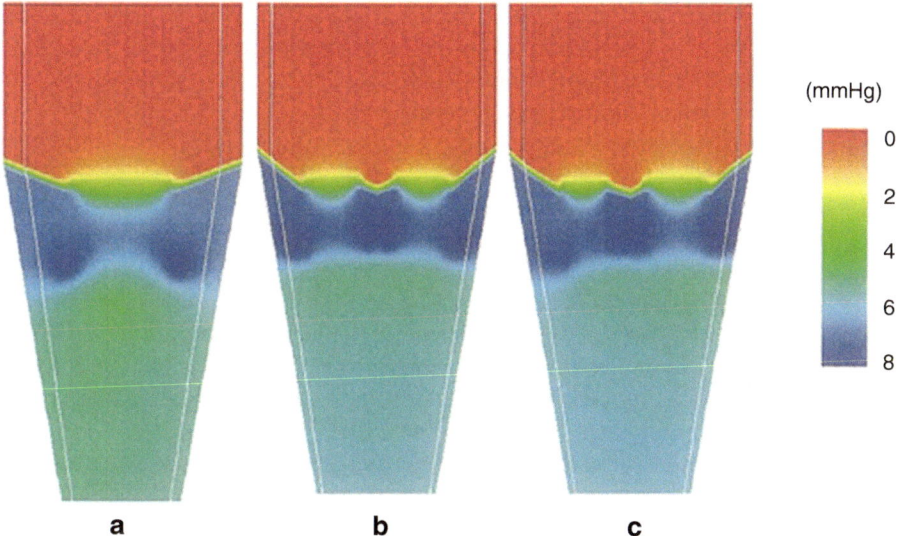

**Fig. 2.3** Pressure colour map for simulations (**a**) single orifice, (**b**) double orifice with equal, and (**c**) unequal areas (Reproduced with permission from [3])

echo-Doppler examination. This was a meaningful example of how the results of a computational model were concretely translated in the all-day clinical practice.

The same results were subsequently confirmed in an in vivo animal model [5, 6]. The excellent very long-term results of the EE technique, which are nowadays available, are the best demonstration that the model was completely adequate and effective in predicting the reliability of the technique in the clinical setting [7].

More recently, the EE procedure opened the way to transcatheter solutions to treat mitral regurgitation. While the computational simulation of the double-orifice repair still represents the basis for the management and decision making in patients receiving the surgical procedure, the same rules apply to the interventional approach.

## 2.2   Evaluation of Residual MR After MitraClip Implantation: An Emerging Issue

Significant residual mitral regurgitation after surgical edge-to-edge is very rare. In the last years, the need for a precise quantification of the residual mitral regurgitation became important after the MitraClip, which is often associated to residual jets, raising the clinical question of how to quantify MR in patients with more than one jet.

In clinical practice, echocardiography plays the leading role in the evaluation of the result after MitraClip implantation by using different parameters for grading MR post-intervention [8]. Residual MR can easily be detected by color Doppler.

However for quantification, it has to be taken into consideration that the area of color jets is larger with multiple jets, which commonly occurs after a MitraClip is implanted (due to the addition of multiple jet areas), than if there is a single jet. This may potentially lead to overestimating residual MR in patients with multiple jets. In vitro studies demonstrated that a fixed regurgitant volume involving multiple jets have a larger jet area than the same total volume from a single jet [9].

The PISA method is not validated for multiple MR jets, nor for the newly created geometry of the MV with two (or even more) orifices, therefore cannot be used to quantify the MR post-procedure.

The summation of two-dimensionally measured venae contracta is not reliable in the presence of multiple jets. However, the direct measurement of the vena contracta area in 3D echocardiography shows potential for the quantification of MR with irregularly shaped vena contracta areas, although further clinical evaluations are required [10].

Computational model may help to answer this question, allowing simulation of residual MR in different clinical and anatomical setting, suggesting the best strategy to quantify multiple residual jet in the context of a double-orifice valve compared to single-orifice valve.

## 2.3    Structural Effects on the MV

One of the potential downsides of the EE technique consists in the extra tensions induced by the stitch on MV leaflets. Limited durability and the risk of suture dehiscence were initially perceived as a critical issue, although rarely seen in clinical practice. The fast expansion of the transcatheter procedures has renovated the interest of clinicians towards this topic. Leaflet rupture and device detachment have been reported after MitraClip, and the underlying mechanism of these complications finds a clear explanation in the results of computational analysis.

In general, the direct measurement of leaflets stresses in complex structure such as the MV is difficult: at best, these can be indirectly estimated from measured strains through the use of constitutive models and numerical techniques. For this reason, experimental studies on this specific aspect were focused on the measurement of the stitch tension, which, due to equilibrium conditions, is transmitted to the leaflets generating stresses [5, 11].

The first finite element analysis of this kind was proposed by Votta et al. [12]. The model provided the first quantification of leaflets stresses following EE repair, and of the influence of suture dimensions, annular dilation, and peak diastolic transmitral pressure. The results suggested a doubled frequency of leaflets mechanical loading after EE as compared to physiological conditions. Independently from other parameters, as the extension of the suture decreased by 50 %, radial stresses decreased both close to the suture and close to the annulus, while circumferential stresses increased next to the suture and decreased in the annular region. Annular dilation (simulated by a 20 % increase in annular diameter) led to massive stress increase regardless of other parameters and interfered significantly with stresses in

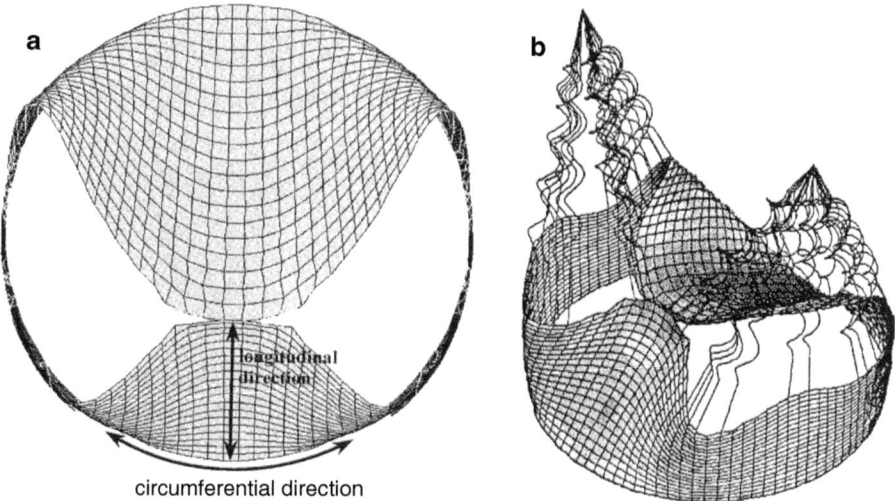

a

b

longitudinal
direction

circumferential direction

**Fig. 2.4** (**a**) Depiction of longitudinal and circumferential directions, (**b**) mitral valve during opening with 15 mmHg applied to the leaflets

the region of the leaflets close to the suture, appearing as the most critical factor for the durability of the repair from a mechanical standpoint (Figs. 2.4 and 2.5). This circumstance may cause repair failure and increase the risk of late tissue degeneration, and may also suggest that the implantation of an annuloplasty device is required in presence of annular dilation.

The outcomes from this modeling, although hampered by several methodologic limitations, have been effectively used to drive clinical practice and decision making, representing another example of how the results of a computational model were concretely translated in the all-day clinical practice. In fact, the surgical EE has been usually associated with annuloplasty in clinical surgical practice, on the basis of these findings. Further clinical series confirmed then this aspect, showing increased repair durability in patients receiving an annuloplasty associated to the edge-to-edge [13].

## 2.4 Structural and Functional Effects of the MitraClip Procedure: A Novel Finite Element Analysis

The latest progress in the story of the EE technique is the transition from the surgical to the percutaneous access, which is currently performed in the real world through the MitraClip system.

Although the MitraClip procedure has been developed to reproduce the surgical procedure, the design of the clip determines specific structural implications: the way the clip interferes with the leaflet at the site of the implant is profoundly different from the surgical sutures. We recently developed a novel analysis of the biomechanical effects of MitraClip implantation (Fig. 2.6), based on image-based finite

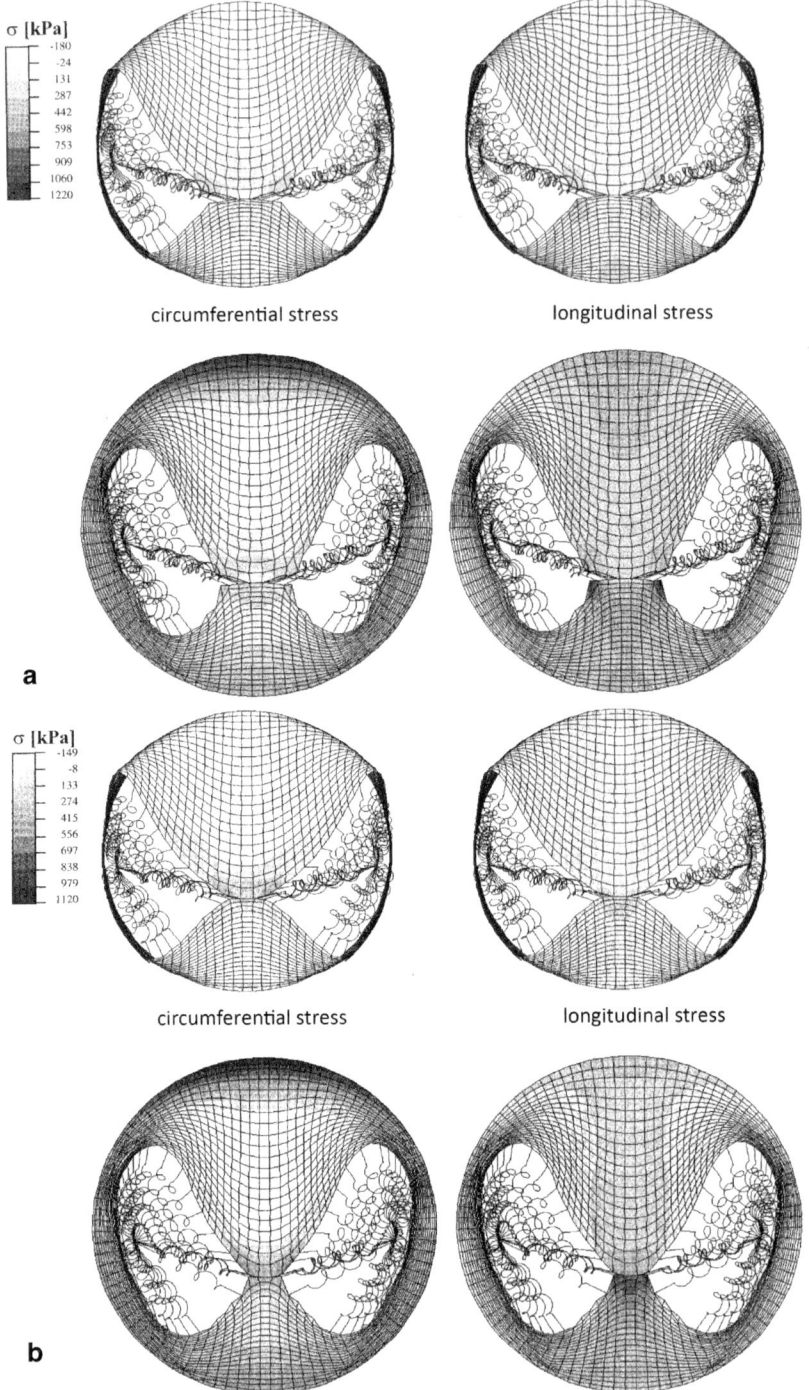

**Fig. 2.5** Circumferential and longitudinal stresses distribution of the closed valve (*above*), and of the closed valve with annular dilation of +20 % (*below*), with 8 mm suture (**a**) and 4 mm suture (**b**)

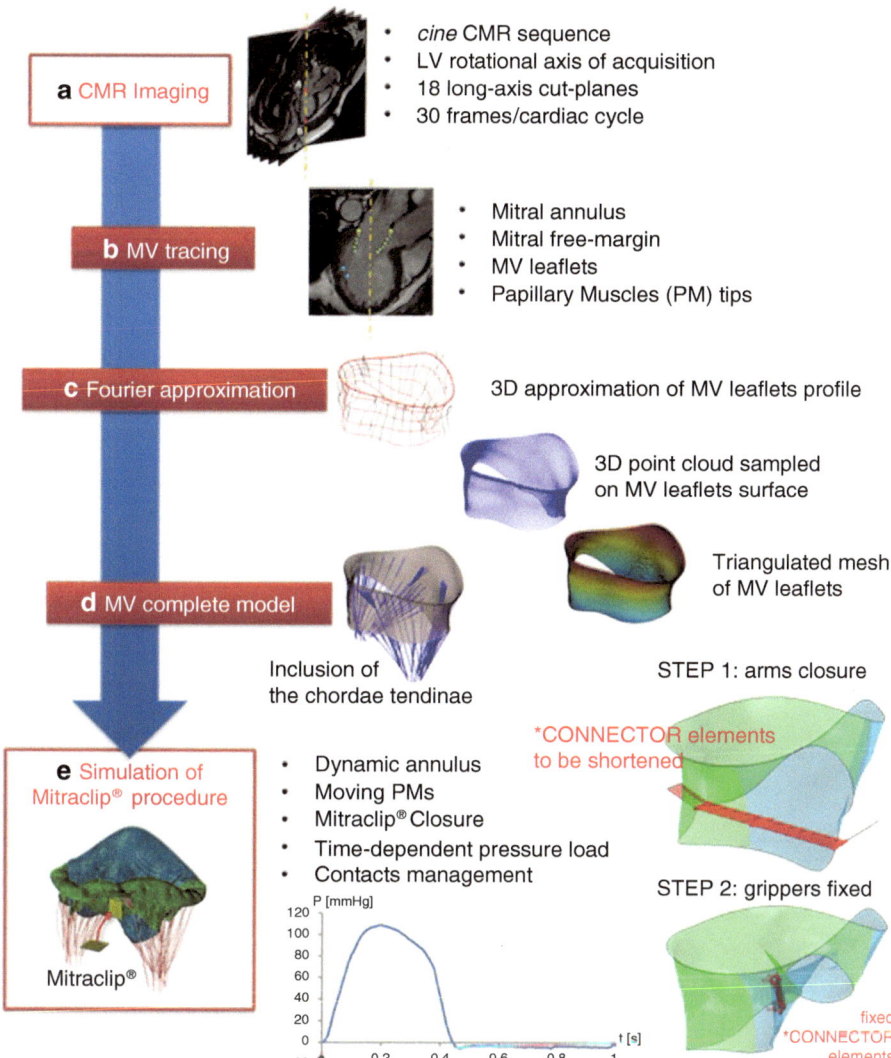

**Fig. 2.6** Computational set-up for the simulation of the MitraClip procedure, including the MitraClip modeling strategy, the dynamic CMR-derived motion of MV annulus and PMs, and the prescribed time-dependent transmitral pressure load, used to simulate a complete cardiac cycle

element modeling [14]. Computational modeling allows to achieve a rather exhaustive simulation of the MitraClip procedure on a real MV pathological scenario, reliably reproducing the approximation of MV leaflets obtained during the procedure [14]. The biomechanical insight provided by a patient-specific finite element analysis may play a key role in order to elucidate the current challenges of the MitraClip percutaneous strategy.

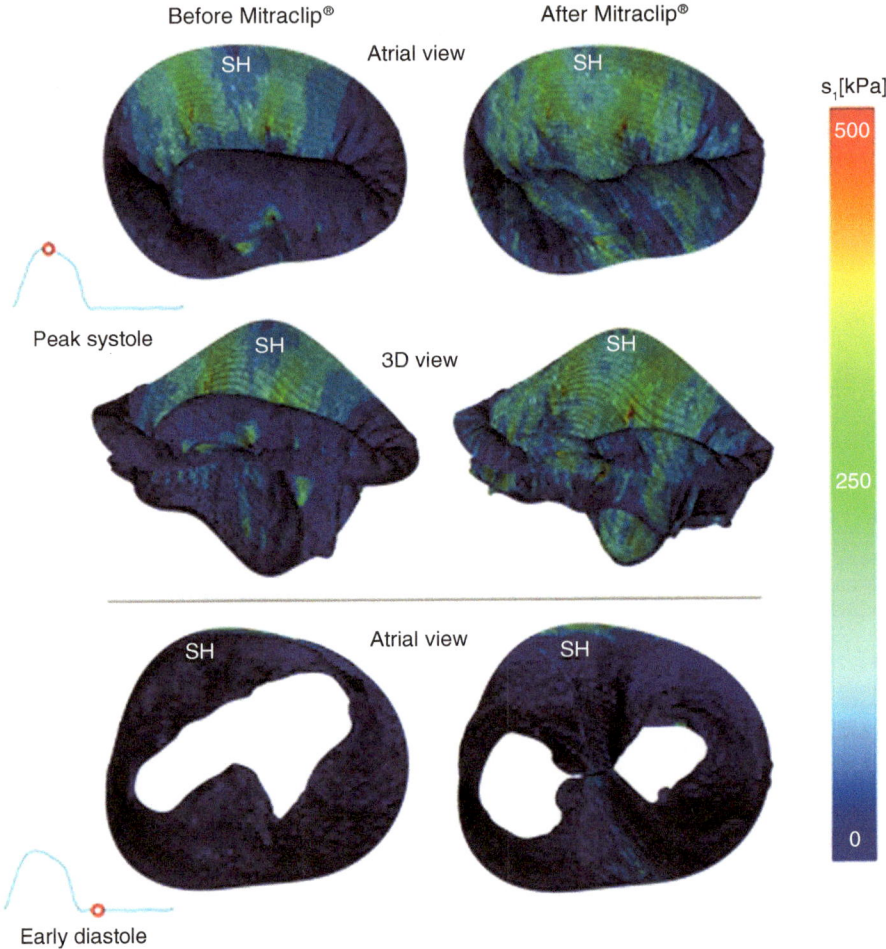

**Fig. 2.7** Maximum principal mechanical stress computed on MV leaflets at peak systole (*upper panel*) and at early diastole (*lower panel*), before and after MitraClip procedure, respectively

MV biomechanics in pathological conditions and following MitraClip procedure have been investigated through computational simulations of a full cardiac cycle.

In each simulation, systolic function could be assessed in terms of leaflet mechanical stresses, systolic coaptation area and coaptation length, which, from a macroscopical point of view, can be considered effective outcome parameters. Diastolic function was evaluated and stresses were computed and the orifice area was quantified in 2D (Fig. 2.7). As result the MitraClip implantation strongly impacted on MV diastolic leaflets configuration reproducing the typical "double orifice" which inherently induces a major reduction in effective orifice area, with respect to preoperative conditions; coaptation length markedly increases to restore a sufficient level of coaptation along the entire posterior leaflet.

MitraClip implantation significantly improved systolic leaflets coaptation, without inducing major alterations in systolic peak stresses.

Future computational modeling approach will include studies to analyze some critical aspects regarding stress distribution after MitraClip implantation, which may help future optimization and improvement of this technology:

(i) Simulation of stress distribution in different clinical scenarios that are currently critical for MitraClip implantation (such as severe functional MR and severe annular dilation or Barlow disease);

(ii) Prediction of leaflets suboptimal grasping between the arms of the device resulting in a periprocedural MitraClip malposition;

(iii) Simulation of anatomy distortion after the implantation of more than one MitraClip devices during the same procedure.

The proposed model will lead to a better definition of the complex interactions between the MV and the MitraClip therapy, the related physiological and pathological hemodynamic conditions, and the outcomes following different approaches. We expect to gain substantial insights about indicators for the prognosis of MR recurrence based on this patient-specific modeling. This understanding is expected to drive a more precise and tailored therapeutic approach to each mitral regurgitation condition, to the development of new and oriented MR therapies, by designing more physiological devices respecting fluid–structure interaction, and will in the end equip the clinician with information and tools for patient-specific therapeutic strategies and timing.

# References

1. de Leval MR, Dubini G, Migliavacca F, Jalali H, Camporini G, Redington A, Pietrabissa R. Use of computational fluid dynamics in the design of surgical procedures: Application to the study of competitive flows in cavo-pulmonary connections. J Thorac Cardiovasc Surg. 1996;111:502–13.
2. Pennati G, Redaelli A, Bellotti M, Ferrazzi E. Computational analysis of the ductus venosus fluid dynamics based on doppler measurements. Ultrasound Med Biol. 1996;22:1017–29.
3. Maisano F, Redaelli A, Pennati G, Fumero R, Torracca L, Alfieri O. The hemodynamic effects of double-orifice valve repair for mitral regurgitation: a 3d computational model. Eur J Cardiothorac Surg. 1999;15:419–25.
4. Redaelli A, Guadagni G, Fumero R, Maisano F, Alfieri O. A computational study of the hemodynamics after "edge-to-edge" mitral valve repair. J Biomech Eng. 2001;123:565–70.
5. Nielsen SL, Timek TA, Lai DT, Daughters GT, Liang D, Hasenkam JM, Ingels NB, Miller DC. Edge-to-edge mitral repair: tension on the approximating suture and leaflet deformation during acute ischemic mitral regurgitation in the ovine heart. Circulation. 2001;104:129–35.
6. Timek TA, Nielsen SL, Liang D, Lai DT, Dagum P, Daughters GT, Ingels Jr NB, Miller DC. Edge-to-edge mitral repair: gradients and three-dimensional annular dynamics in vivo during inotropic stimulation. Eur J Cardiothorac Surg. 2001;19:431–7.
7. De Bonis M, Lapenna E, Taramasso M, La Canna G, Buzzatti N, Pappalardo F, Alfieri O. Very long-term durability of the edge-to-edge repair for isolated anterior mitral leaflet prolapse: up to 21 years of clinical and echocardiographic results. J Thorac Cardiovasc Surg. 2014;148:2027–32.

8. Wunderlich NC, Siegel RJ. Peri-interventional echo assessment for the mitraclip procedure. Eur Heart J Cardiovasc Imaging. 2013;14:935–49.
9. Lin BA, Forouhar AS, Pahlevan NM, Anastassiou CA, Grayburn PA, Thomas JD, Gharib M. Color doppler jet area overestimates regurgitant volume when multiple jets are present. J Am Soc Echocardiogr. 2010;23:993–1000.
10. Gruner C, Herzog B, Bettex D, Felix C, Datta S, Greutmann M, Gaemperli O, Muggler SA, Tanner FC, Gruenenfelder J, Corti R, Biaggi P. Quantification of mitral regurgitation by real time three-dimensional color doppler flow echocardiography pre- and post-percutaneous mitral valve repair. Echocardiography. 2014.
11. Timek TA, Nielsen SL, Lai DT, Tibayan F, Liang D, Daughters GT, Beineke P, Hastie T, Ingels Jr NB, Miller DC. Mitral annular size predicts Alfieri stitch tension in mitral edge-to-edge repair. J Heart Valve Dis. 2004;13:165–73.
12. Votta E, Maisano F, Soncini M, Redaelli A, Montevecchi FM, Alfieri O. 3-d computational analysis of the stress distribution on the leaflets after edge-to-edge repair of mitral regurgitation. J Heart Valve Dis. 2002;11:810–22.
13. Maisano F, Caldarola A, Blasio A, De Bonis M, La Canna G, Alfieri O. Midterm results of edge-to-edge mitral valve repair without annuloplasty. J Thorac Cardiovasc Surg. 2003;126:1987–97.
14. Sturla F, Redaelli A, Puppini G, Onorati F, Faggian G, Votta E. Functional and biomechanical effects of the edge-to-edge repair in the setting of mitral regurgitation: consolidated knowledge and novel tools to gain insight into its percutaneous implementation. Cardiovasc Eng Tech. 2014;1–24.

# Technical Aspects: Sternotomy and Minimally Invasive Approaches

**3**

Andrea Fumero and Michele De Bonis

## 3.1 Introduction

The edge-to-edge (EE) technique is a method to treat mitral valve (MV) regurgitation by suturing the edges of the leaflets at the site of regurgitation. Although the method is technically simple, its application should follow precise rules to avoid complications and to ensure durable results.

In terms of surgical approaches, several different solutions have been described from the beginning of mitral valve surgery. A left thoracotomy was the technique of choice in the pioneers' era, when mitral commissurotomy was performed with digital dilatation. Subsequently the median sternotomy became the standard approach. Nowadays a right antero-lateral minithoracotomy is often used.

The first EE repair was performed through a median sternotomy in 1991, while the first right minithoracotomy approach was adopted shortly later.

In this chapter we describe the surgical technique for central and commissural EE repair by sternotomy or right minithoracotomy.

## 3.2 Approaches

### 3.2.1 Median Sternotomy

A complete median sternotomy is performed trough a skin incision starting 2–4 cm below the jugular notch and ending 3 cm before the xiphoid process (Fig. 3.1). The pericardium is opened longitudinally and transversally on the diaphragmatic folder, especially on the left side to join the heart apex. The right side of the pericardium is fixed

A. Fumero, MD • M. De Bonis, MD, PhD (✉)
Department of Cardiac Surgery, IRCCS San Raffaele University Hospital,
Via Olgettina 60, Milan 20132, Italy
e-mail: fumero.andrea@hsr.it; debonis.michele@hsr.it

© Springer International Publishing Switzerland 2015
O. Alfieri et al. (eds.), *Edge-to-Edge Mitral Repair: From a Surgical to a Percutaneous Approach*, DOI 10.1007/978-3-319-19893-4_3

**Fig. 3.1** Median sternotomy

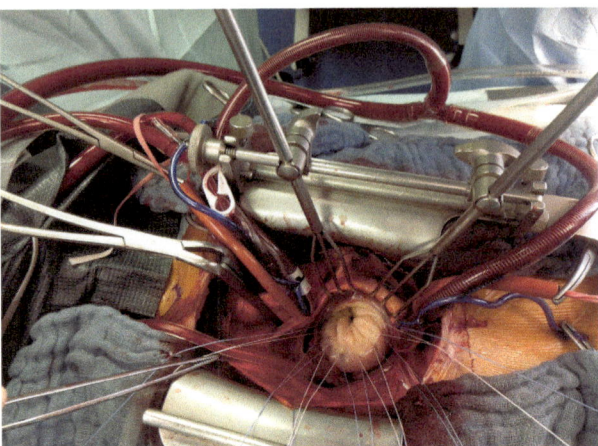

**Fig. 3.2** Mitral valve
exposure through median
sternotomy

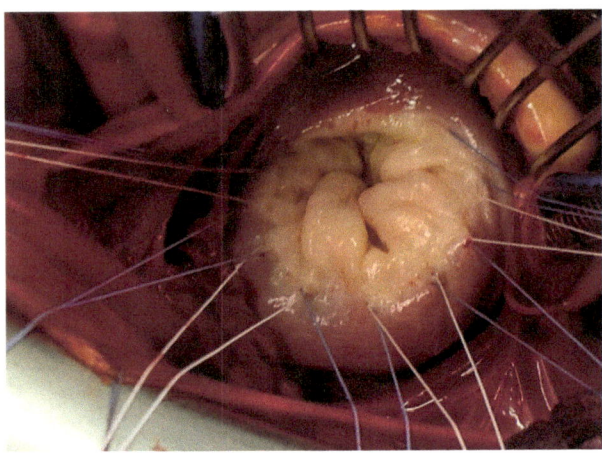

to the skin with three stay sutures, while the left side is not suspended. This generates a
rotation of the heart towards the left, leading to a better exposure of the left atrium. The
ascending aorta and the inferior and superior venae cavae are cannulated for cardiopulmonary bypass (CPB). Moreover a single purse string is positioned on the aortic root for
a Y cannula to administer cardioplegia and venting. Before CPB is started, the inter-
atrial groove is dissected. On hypothermic CPB, the aorta is cross-clamped and the heart
arrested by antegrade cold cardioplegia delivery (Custodiol®). The left atrium is opened
longitudinally in the inter-atrial groove from the roof to the proximity of the inferior
vena cava and the mitral valve is exposed with a Cosgrove retractor (Fig. 3.2). A vent is
positioned into the left atrium through the right superior pulmonary vein. The valve is
then assessed by using a forceps and a hook. Depending on the MR etiology, annular
stitches with 2-0 Ticron® are placed only in the posterior annulus from trigone to trigone
(degenerative) or along its entire circumference (functional), starting from the anterolateral commisure counterclockwise. The edge-to-edge suture is then performed.

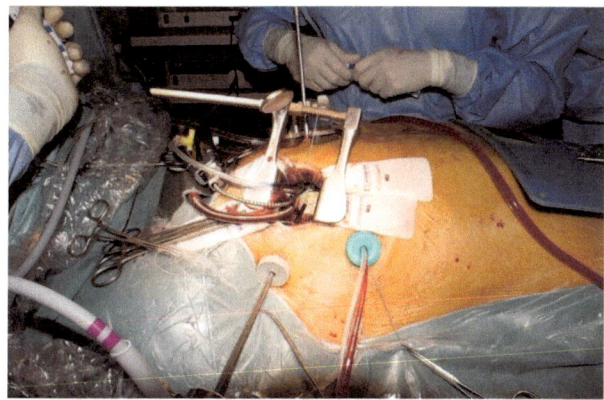

**Fig. 3.3**  Right minithoracotomy surgical field

Once the repair is complete, valve competence is tested by filling the left ventricle with saline or cardioplegic solution and the patient is rewarmed. A left ventricular vent is positioned through the mitral valve for dearing and the left atrium is closed. A Valsalva maneuver is performed and the aortic cross-clamp removed. After weaning from CPB, the mitral valve is checked with trans-esophageal echo and protamine is eventually given.

## 3.2.2  Minithoracotomy

The patient is positioned in a 30° left side rotation. The right femoral artery is marked at the inguinal folding. The jugular notch and the xiphoid process are also marked for emergent sternotomy. The III° and IV° intercostals spaces are marked in their right parasternal portions. Femoral artery and vein are exposed with a transverse incision 2 cm higher than the inguinal folding. Two 5-0 prolene purse strings are used for Seldinger cannulation of the femoral artery and vein. In men, a 7–9 cm skin incision is performed in correspondence of the III° or IV° intercostal space, starting 2 cm lateral to the median clavear line (Fig. 3.3). In women, the mammary groove is preferred for the surgical cut for cosmetic reasons. A blunt dissection between pectoral and intercostals muscles is performed to reach the proper intercostal space. As a general rule, if there are no contraindications to femoral artery cannulation and retrograde perfusion, a IV° intercostal space minithoracotomy is preferred. On the other hand, if peripheral arterial cannulation and retrograde perfusion is not recommended for the small size of the artery, presence of abdominal or thoracic aortic aneurism or aortic thrombi, a minithoracotomy in the III° intercostal space allows a direct cannulation of the ascending aorta (Fig. 3.4). A soft tissue retractor is used with or without a small rib retractor.

A 5.5 mm trocar is placed in the same intercostal space chosen for the surgical access about 12 cm below the lower end of the skin incision. This port will be used for the insertion of a 5 mm 30° camera. Similarly, a left atrium retractor is inserted through the intercostal space about 10–12 cm above the superior end of the skin

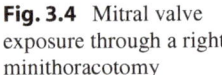

**Fig. 3.4** Mitral valve
exposure through a right
minithoracotomy

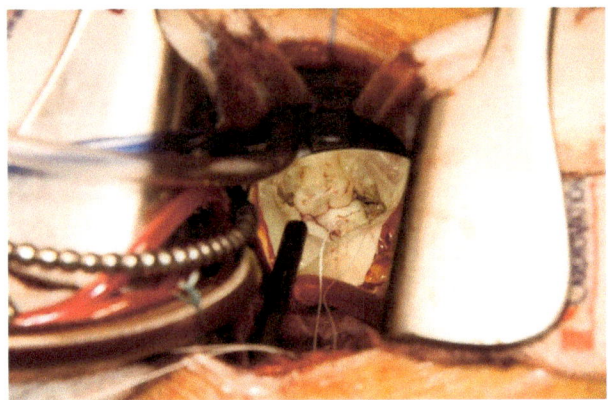

incision. Finally another trocar is placed two intercostal spaces lower than the one
used for the minithoracotomy incision to inflate 1.5 L/min of $CO_2$ and to insert the
left atrial vent. The pericardium is then opened 2–3 cm above the phrenic nerve.
Two single pericardial stay-sutures (corresponding to the superior and inferior right
pulmonary veins) are used for exposure.

At this point three different cannulation strategies can be adopted:

1. *Total peripheral cannulation*

   Heparin is administrated and the femoral artery and vein are cannulated with
   Seldinger technique. An 18 or 20 french arterial cannula (Medtronic Eopa®) is
   inserted through a single 5-0 prolene purse string. With the same technique, a
   femoral vein cannula (Edwards QD® 22 or 25) is advanced under echo view into
   the superior vena cava. To facilitate this maneuver a Trendelemburg position can
   be used.

2. *Femoral vein cannulation and aortic cannulation*

   This solution can be adopted whenever the cannulation of the femoral artery
   is unsuitable or a retrograde perfusion is contraindicated. Heparin is administrated and femoral vein cannulation is performed as previously described or,
   alternatively, by using a totally percutaneous approach with Seldinger technique
   without any surgical cut down. Two 4-0 prolene purse strings are prepared on the
   lateral surface of the distal ascending aorta and an Edwards® StraightShot 23 F
   aortic cannula is put in place.

3. *Jugular and femoral vein cannulation*

   Whenever the opening of the right atrium is required (as in concomitant tricuspid repair or atrial fibrillation ablation), the superior vena cava can be
   percutaneously cannulated through the right internal jugular vein with a Maquet
   HLS ® arterial armed cannula 15 or 17 french. Once this cannula is in place, the
   pericardium is opened and a femoral vein cannula (Medtronic DPL® 28 french or
   Edwards VFEM® 24 french) is advanced in the inferior vena cava and positioned
   just before the right atrium entrance. For arterial cannulation the same strategies
   previously described can be associated (femoral artery or ascending aorta).

Once cannulation has been performed, the interatrial groove is gently dissected and CPB is started. When the heart is empty, a U 4-0 prolene suture with pledgets is saw on the lateral face of the aorta and a long aortic needle cannula is placed to administer cardioplegia and for venting. A Cygnet® flexible aortic clamp (Novare Surgical Systems, Inc., Cupertino, CA) is used to clamp the aorta through the mini-thoracotomy. The left atrium is then opened, the mitral valve is exposed and the surgical repair is carried out. If the water test is satisfactory, a ventricular vent is positioned through the mitral valve and the left atrium is closed. A Valsalva maneuver is performed for deairing, a single epicardial temporary bipolar pacing wire is positioned on the right ventricle, aortic cross-clamp is removed and weaning from CPB is achieved. Finally the result of the edge-to-edge repair is checked by transesophageal echo.

## 3.3  Technical Aspects of Leaflet Repair

As far as the technical aspects of the EE technique is concerned, the first step is represented by a careful valve analysis in order to confirm the etiology of the disease and the mechanism of regurgitation. Annular sutures for prosthetic ring implantation can be placed to obtain a better view.

Unlike the traditional repair techniques, which realize an anatomical reconstruction of the diseased valve, the basic concept behind the EE approach is that the competence of the mitral valve can be effectively restored with a "functional" rather than an "anatomical" repair [1]. The location of the jet of MR, as identified by echocardiography, is particularly important because exactly at that level the free edge of one leaflet is sutured to the corresponding edge of the opposing leaflet to restore valve competence. When the regurgitation originates in the central part of the valve, the EE produces a mitral valve with a double orifice configuration (double orifice repair). On the other hand, when mitral insufficiency occurs in proximity of a commissure, the EE leads to a surgical closure of the commissure ("paracommissural EE repair"). Under these circumstances, the mitral valve will have a single orifice with a relatively smaller area compared to the preoperative value. The suture has to be placed exactly in correspondence of the regurgitant jet and has to be as short as possible in order to eliminate MR without inducing stenosis. Valve distortion has to be carefully avoided as well. A ring annuloplasty should be used and a final mitral valve area $\geq 2.5$ cm$^2$ should be left in normal size patients.

### 3.3.1  Central Edge-to-Edge

If the valve lesion is located at the middle of one or both leaflets, the EE suture generates a double orifice valve (Fig. 3.5) [2]. In most cases of degenerative mitral regurgitation, a 4-0 polypropylene suture (double armed prolene SH-1) is usually appropriate, since leaflets are thick and redundant. A 5-0 polypropylene suture may be preferable in case of thin tissues. Pledgets are rarely necessary. If there is a flail

**Fig. 3.5** Double-orifice
edge-to-edge repair

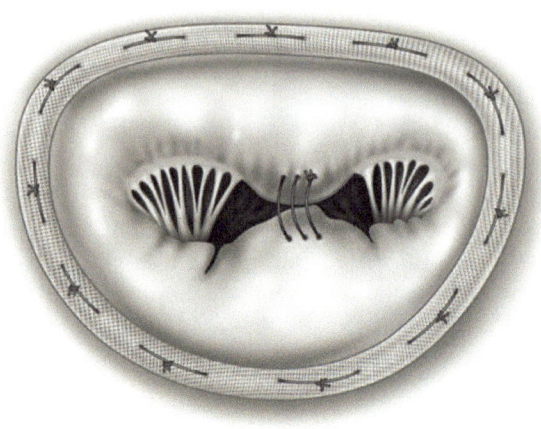

**Fig. 3.6** Exposure of the
subvalvular apparatus to
identify the middle segment
of the anterior leaflet

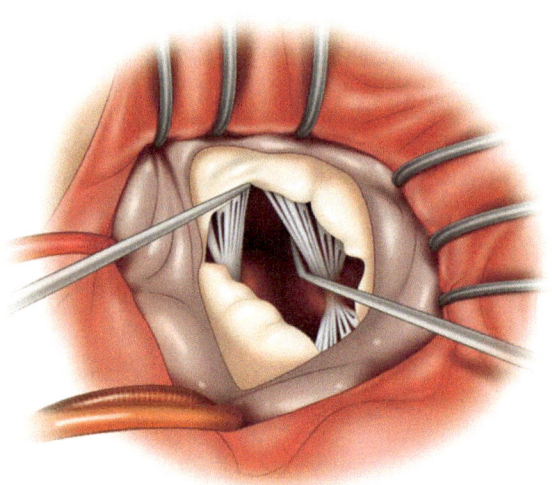

leaflet, the stitch may include the flail segment. More often, however, particularly in bileaflet prolapse due to Barlow's disease, there are no flail leaflets, but all portions of the valve prolapse. In this case, the stitch is positioned exactly at the "anatomical middle" of the valve [3]. The anatomical middle of the valve can be defined as the point where the subvalvar structures converge in the middle of the anterior and posterior leaflets. This point divides the valve into two symmetric halves, each one connected to one papillary muscle. The convergence of the chordae coming from the anterior and posterior papillary muscles is inspected with a nerve hook (Fig. 3.6) and the suture is passed deeply into the anterior leaflet body at this site (Figs. 3.7 and 3.8). The same is done for the posterior leaflet (Fig. 3.9). Once the first stitch

**Fig. 3.7** The center of the middle scallop of the anterior leaflet (A2) has been identified and the first stitch is going to be placed at that level

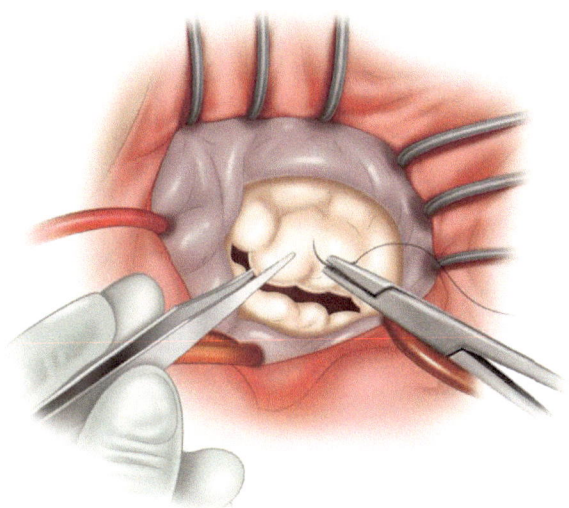

**Fig. 3.8** The first stitch has been passed through the middle scallop of the anterior leaflet

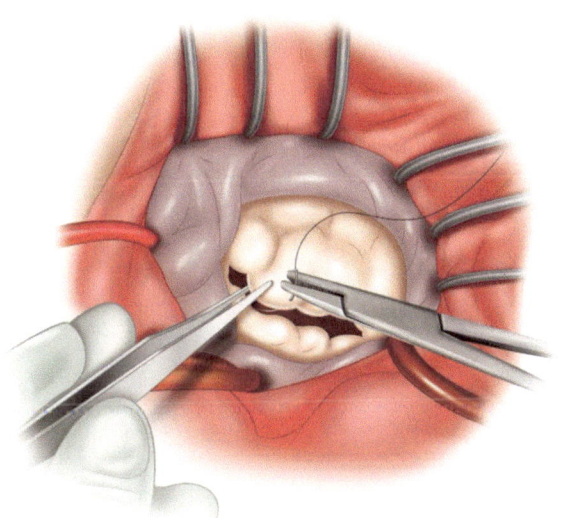

has been passed, symmetry of the suture is checked (Figs. 3.10 and 3.11) and the suture is run towards the commissures as needed (Figs. 3.12 and 3.13). Two rows of suture are placed, the first is continuous mattress and the second is over-and-over continuous suture. Stitch depth is approximately 0.5–1 cm from the free edge of the leaflets: the more redundancy is present, the deeper the stitch, and wider the suture. As a rule, the width of this suture should be minimized to decrease the risk of valvular stenosis. If valve prolapse and leaflet redundancy is severe, a wider suture,

**Fig. 3.9** The first stitch has
been passed through the
middle scallops of the
anterior leaflet and posterior
leaflet

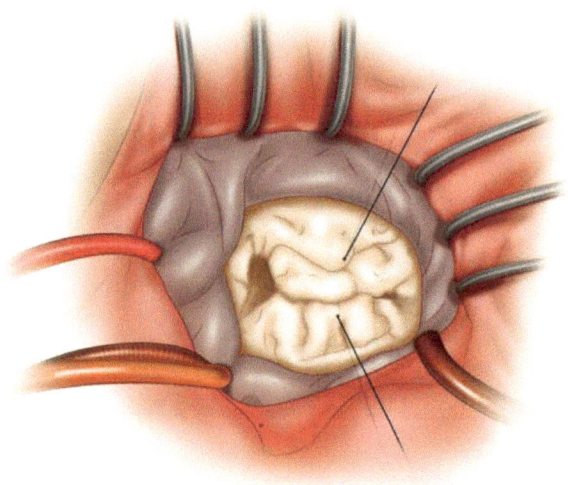

**Fig. 3.10** The orifices are
checked

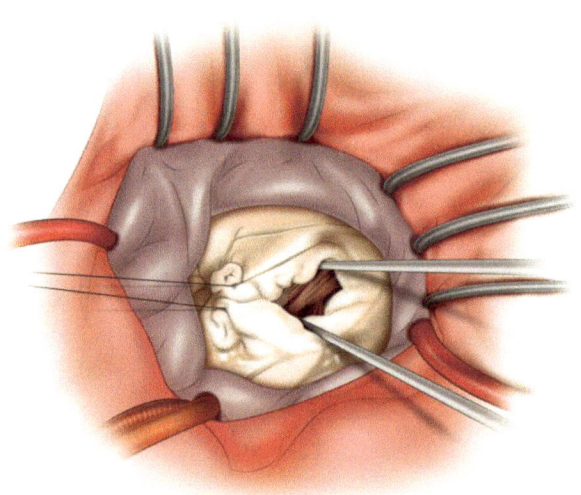

connecting the whole P2 free edge to the opposing A2, may be necessary (Figs. 3.12
and 3.13). This solution should be reserved only for those cases with a very large
preoperative area. If there is any doubt regarding the post-repair valve area, the
valve orifices should be probed with Hegar dilators to assess orifice areas. The total
valve area should be greater than 2.5 cm$^2$ Annuloplasty is necessary to remodel and
to reduce the size of the annulus. Ring size is chosen as usual, by measuring the
intertrigonal distance and the anterior leaflet surface area. In double orifice repair
large rings are usually needed.

**Fig. 3.11** The overall aspect of the mitral valve is checked to exclude geometric distortion

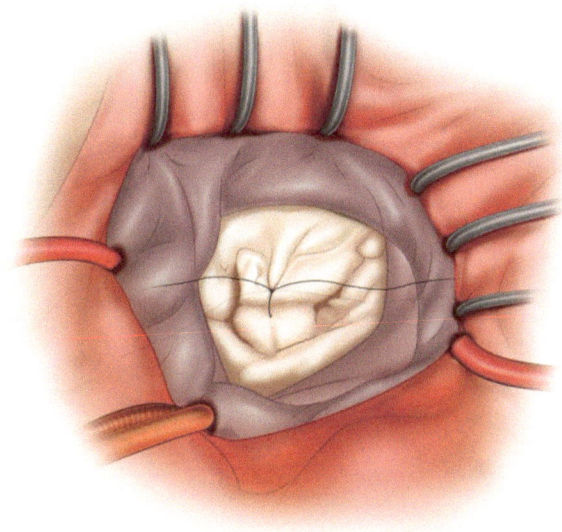

**Fig. 3.12** The edge-to-edge suture of A2 and P2 is completed (systolic view)

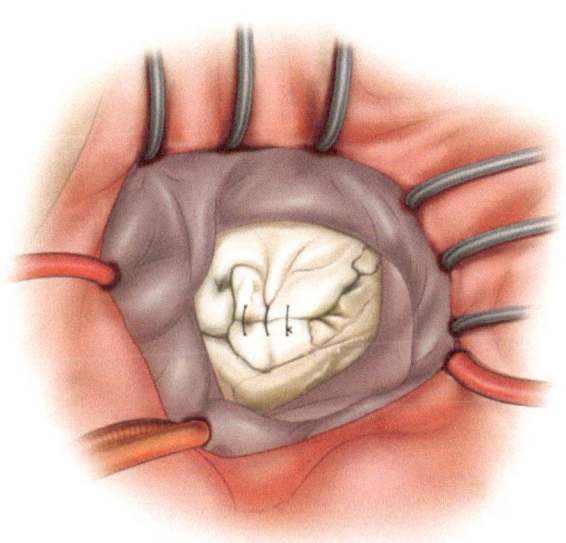

Intraoperative post-repair TEE is mandatory to exclude residual regurgitation and valve stenosis. Valve area may be assessed by Doppler methods [4]. However we mostly rely on planimetric valve area, assessed in the transgastric, short-axis view of the mitral valve.

**Fig. 3.13** The edge-to-edge suture of A2 and P2 is completed (diastolic view)

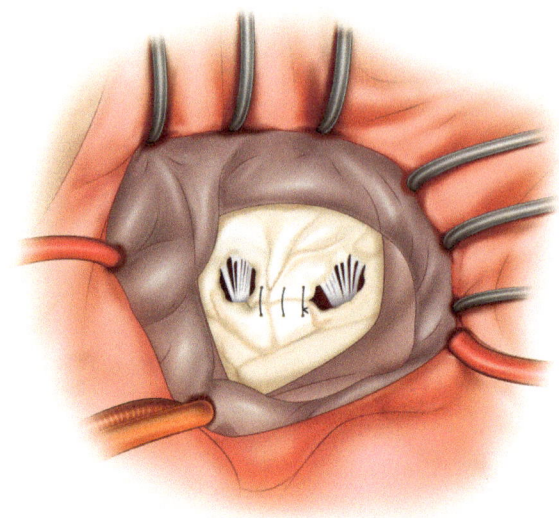

**Fig. 3.14** Paracommissural edge-to-edge repair

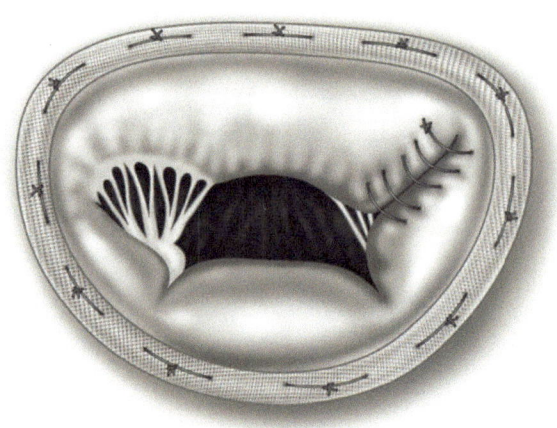

### 3.3.2   Paracommissural Edge-to-Edge

When mitral insufficiency occurs in proximity of a commissure, elongated or ruptured chordae of the anterior and/or posterior leaflet are typically found at this level. In this case, the application of the EE technique leads to a surgical closure of the commissure ("paracommissural EE repair") [5–7] (Fig. 3.14). The normal chordae on one or both leaflets adjacent to the area of prolapse are identified to mark the limits of the commissural closure. The entire prolapsing commissural region is then closed by suturing the free edge of the anterior leaflet to the free edge of the posterior leaflet with a 4.0 or 5.0 polypropylene buttress suture followed by a continuous running suture. According to the location of the regurgitant jet and the site of prolapse identified intraoperatively, the EE suture is performed at the posteromedial or anterolateral commissure. As for the central EE, it is essential to respect the symmetry of the valve and avoid distortion. The mitral valve will eventually have a single orifice with a relatively smaller area compared to the preoperative value. Prosthetic ring annuloplasty is then added to complete the repair. If necessary, the residual orifice area can be measured with the use of Hegar dilators. However, according to our long-term results, this technique does not cause any significant restriction as confirmed by the low transvalvular pressure gradients recorded immediately after surgery and at the last echocardiographic follow-up examination [6, 7].

## References

1. Maisano F, Torracca L, Oppizzi M, et al. The edge-to-edge technique: a simplified method to correct mitral insufficiency. Eur J Cardiothorac Surg. 1998;13:240–6.
2. Alfieri O, Maisano F, De Bonis M, et al. The double-orifice technique in mitral valve repair: a simple solution for complex problems. J Thorac Cardiovasc Surg. 2001;122:674–81.
3. Maisano F, Schreuder JJ, Oppizzi M, Fiorani B, Fino C, Alfieri O. The double-orifice technique as a standardized approach to treat mitral regurgitation due to severe myxomatous disease: surgical technique. Eur J Cardiothorac Surg. 2000;17:201–5.
4. Maisano F, Redaelli A, Pennati G, Fumero R, Torracca L, Alfieri O. The hemodynamic effects of double-orifice valve repair for mitral regurgitation: a 3D computational model. Eur J Cardiothorac Surg. 1999;15:419–25.
5. Gillinov AM, Shortt KG, Cosgrove 3rd DM. Commissural closure for repair of mitral commissural prolapse. Ann Thorac Surg. 2005;80:1135–6.
6. Lapenna E, De Bonis M, Sorrentino F, La Canna G, Grimaldi A, Torracca L, et al. Commissural closure for the treatment of commissural mitral valve prolapse or flail. J Heart Valve Dis. 2008;17:261–6.
7. De Bonis M, Lapenna E, Taramasso M, Pozzoli A, La Canna G, Calabrese MC, Alfieri O. Is commissural closure associated with mitral annuloplasty a durable technique for the treatment of mitral regurgitation? A long-term (≤15 years) clinical and echocardiographic study. J Thorac Cardiovasc Surg. 2014;147(6):1900–6.

# Is There a Role for the Edge-to-Edge Technique in Robotic Valve Mitral Repair?

W. Randolph Chitwood Jr.

## 4.1 Background

Robotic techniques have evolved as a precise way to repair mitral valves through the least invasive incisions. The advanced visualization and operative ergonomics of the daVinci™ robotic surgical system provides a new vista for surgeons performing complex repairs. daVinci™ system robotic mitral valve repairs have been done in the United States since the year 2000 [1, 2]. Since then our robotic team has performed over 925 robotic mitral valve repairs with excellent results [3]. Other centers have validated the use of robotics for mitral repairs and have achieved equally excellent outcomes [4, 5].

Simplified mitral repair techniques now include the edge-to-edge (EE) leaflet repair, which since 1991 Alfieri has proven to be efficacious [6–8]. This method has been shown to have excellent long-term outcomes in patients with both simple or complex degenerative mitral disease. In many instances anterior leaflet repairs have been less reproducible with other techniques, such as resections, chordal shortening, and chordal transpositions. Bileaflet prolapse remains additionally challenging for many surgeons. Prolonged aortic cross clamp times have been associated with bileaflet prolapse repairs. Thus, the EE technique has a great potential in both minimally invasive robotic and invasive mitral repairs that tend to have longer perfusion and arrest times.

The question,

"Is there a role for the edge-to-edge technique in robotic valve mitral repair?" – the answer is YES.

W.R. Chitwood Jr., MD
Department of Cardiovascular Sciences, The Brody School of Medicine, East Carolina Heart Institute, East Carolina University, 115 Heart Drive, Greenville, NC 27834, USA
e-mail: chitwoodw@ecu.edu

© Springer International Publishing Switzerland 2015
O. Alfieri et al. (eds.), *Edge-to-Edge Mitral Repair: From a Surgical to a Percutaneous Approach*, DOI 10.1007/978-3-319-19893-4_4

| **Table 4.1** Robotic mitral surgery exclusion criteria | Previous right thoracotomy |
|---|---|
| | Severe liver dysfunction |
| | Bleeding disorders |
| | Pulmonary hypertension (fixed PAS >60 Torr) |
| | Significant aortic valve disease |
| | Coronary artery disease requiring surgery |
| | Recent myocardial ischemia (<30 days) |
| | Recent stroke (<30 days) |
| | Severely calcified mitral valve annulus |

## 4.2    Patient Selection

All patients with isolated degenerative mitral valve disease are considered for a robotic mitral repair. Table 4.1 lists contraindications for using robotics in mitral valve surgery. In patients with severe peripheral vascular disease, we cannulate the axillary artery for cardiopulmonary perfusion. In those over 40 years old, and/or with a strong family history and/or symptoms of coronary disease, angiography is performed; although often we use computed tomographic angiography as a screening test. Patients with poor lung function undergo preoperative pulmonary testing to ascertain whether they will tolerate single lung ventilation. In the presence of severe fixed pulmonary hypertension, we tend to use a sternotomy to provide optimal right ventricular protection.

Although the EE technique has not been our main robotic valve repair strategy, we have used the edge-to-edge robotic technique to correct: (1) bileaflet prolapse (Barlow's disease) and/or severe anterior leaflet prolapse in elderly patients (>75 years old), (2) high-risk patients who require short perfusion times because of multiple comorbidities, (3) commissural prolapse, (4) elderly patients with complete (trigone-to-trigone) annular calcification, (5) refractory post repair systolic anterior motion (SAM), (6) SAM associated with idiopathic hypertrophic sub-aortic stenosis, and (7) residual leaks after another technique repair.

## 4.3    Echocardiographic Planning

### 4.3.1    Pre-repair

Three-dimensional (3-D) trans-esophageal (TEE) studies provide ideal definition of valve pathology and assessment of post-repair flow dynamics. We echo measure all leaflet segments with particular attention to the length of $A_2$ as well as to the height of each posterior scallop ($P_1$, $P_2$, $P_3$). Any level of prolapse is determined for each leaflet scallop. With the EE technique it is important to determine the exact sites and directions of regurgitant jets. Regions of leaflet restriction or commissural malcoaptation should be identified. If the aortic and mitral valve planar angle is significantly less than 120° (especially in the presence of long $A_2$ and $P_2$ scallops) a greater chance of post-repair anterior leaflet systolic anterior motion (SAM) exists. Finally, the annular diameter, outflow tract septal thickness, and coaptation point to septal (C Sept) distances are measured. We have determined previously that the echocardiographic, direct linear, and annuloplasty band/ring sizer measurements of $A_2$ correlate closely. Thus, we rely on TEE measurements to select the annuloplasty prosthesis size.

### 4.3.2 Post-repair

After an edge-to-edge leaflet repair, an echocardiographic trans-valvular Doppler pressure gradient must be determined to define any residual stenosis. Moreover, the post-repair diastolic valve area of both orifices should be defined by echo planimetry. The post-repair pressure gradient relates to the sum of both orifice areas and should be equivalent to that of a single orifice valve.

## 4.4 The daVinci ™ Robotic Surgical System

The da Vinci™ SI HD (high-definition) surgical system used by our group was commercialized in 2009. A new daVinci XI™ has been approved recently by the FDA but has not been proven in cardiac surgery as of this publication. Both the daVinci SI™ and XI™ are comprised of an operating console, an electronic vision cart, and a surgical instrument cart. Figure 4.1 shows the overall operating room arrangement with end-effector instruments used in robotic mitral valve surgery. The surgical cart should be positioned along the left side of the patient with the over arching instrument arms entering the right chest (Fig. 4.2).

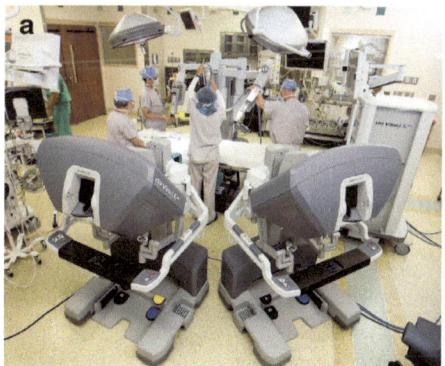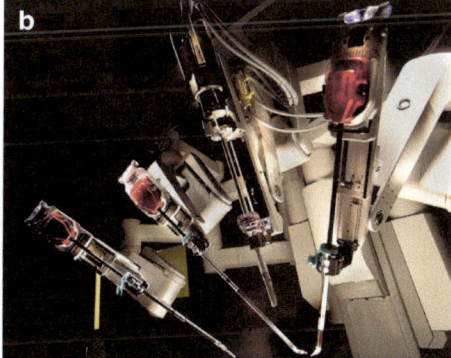

**Fig. 4.1** (**a**) Robotic operating room and instrument cart: The operating room for robotic mitral valve surgery is generally arranged in this fashion. (**b**) The surgical cart is comprised of three instrument arms with end-effector tips. The fourth arm is reserved for the dynamic intra-atrial retractor. The high-definition 3-D camera arm is also shown (With permission from [9])

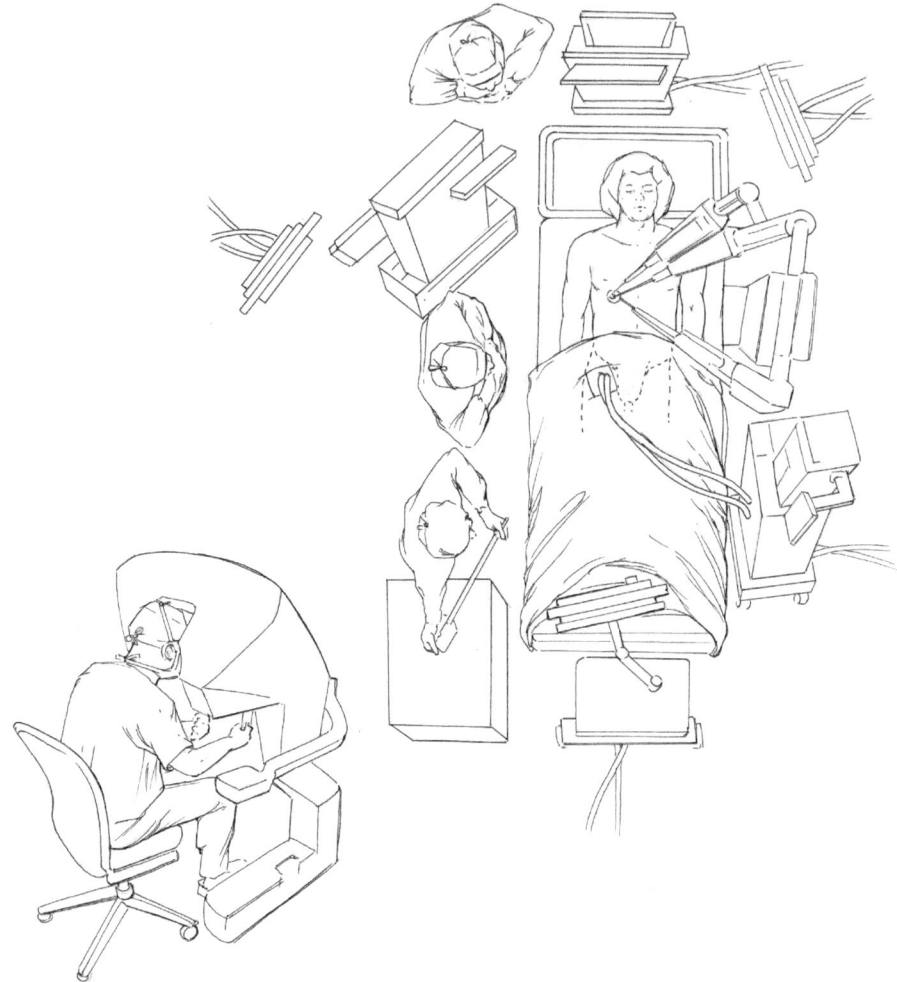

**Fig. 4.2** Operating room set-up: The position of the surgical instrument cart, vision cart, and operative console during robotic mitral valve surgery (With permission from [9])

Individual instrument trocars are inserted through specific intercostal spaces shown in Fig. 4.3. After the two instrument arms, the 3-D camera, and the dynamic retractor have been inserted, the surgeon works from two hand driven sensors that transmit digital instructions to the instrument end effectors. A clutching mechanism enables readjustment of surgeon's hand-positions to maintain an optimal ergonomic attitude with respect to the visual field. The robotic end-effectors have seven degrees of ergonomic freedom that allow surgeons ideal dexterity with both dominant and non-dominant hands (Fig. 4.4).

We use four EndoWrist ™ instruments to perform all robotic mitral repairs (Fig. 4.5). To grasp thickened myxomatous leaflet tissue, we prefer Resano (8-mm)

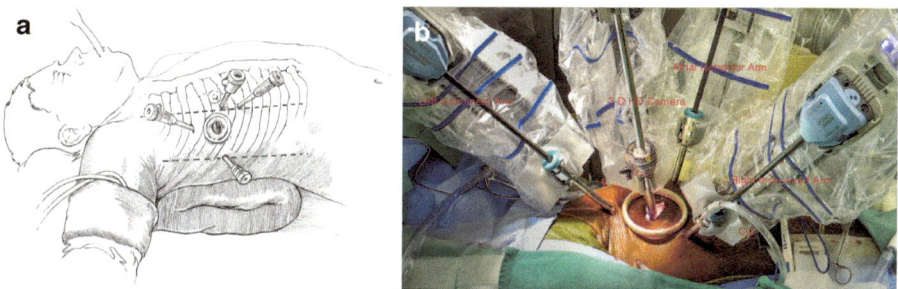

**Fig. 4.3** (**a, b**) Placement of robotic instrument trocars: Instrument arms are inserted through trocars placed in the 3rd (left arm) and 5th (right arm) intercostal spaces (ICS). The camera port is inserted through either an anterior 4th ICS trocar or the 4-cm 4th ICS working port (mini-thoracotomy). The dynamic retractor is placed through a sub-mammary 5th ICS trocar inserted in the mid-clavicular line (With permission from [9])

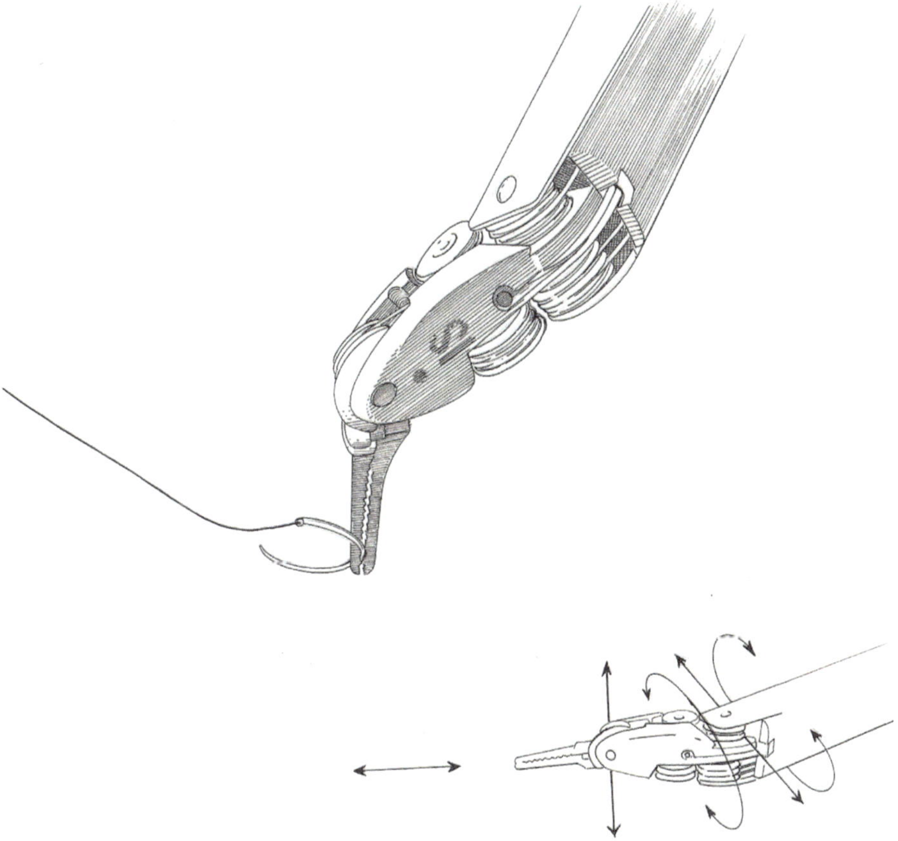

**Fig. 4.4** Robotic instrument "Wrist": The instrument arm and wristed end effectors are able to move forward/backward, up/down, and left/right in combination with rotation about three perpendicular axes, or pitch, yaw, and roll (With permission from [9])

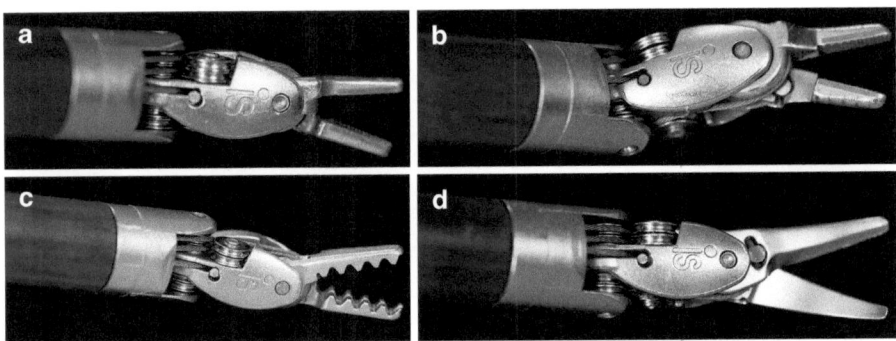

**Fig. 4.5** (**a–d**) Robotic instrument tips (end-effectors): (**a**) Large needle holders. (**b**) Suture-cut™ Needle holders. (**c**) Resano tissue forceps. (**d**) Curved scissors (With permission from [9])

Endowrist ™ forceps. Most sutures are placed using large SutureCut™ Endowrist™ needle drivers. These have great gripping power, especially when angling the needles, and have a suture-cutting surface along the posterior portion of the instrument. Large non-cutting needle drivers are used to remove annular calcium when suturing with PTFE material. Curved Endowrist™ scissors are optimal for all types of mitral valve repairs. The dynamic left atrial retractor provides ideal mitral valve exposure and is easy to reposition.

## 4.5    Preparation and Operative Conduct

### 4.5.1    Anesthesia and Cannulation

Our cardiopulmonary bypass (CPB) cannulation, perfusion, and myocardial protection techniques have been published in detail [9]. With the patient in the supine position, either a double lumen endotracheal tube or bronchial blocker is inserted. Then, the 3-D trans-esophageal echocardiographic probe is positioned and detailed studies are completed. A thermo-dilution Swan–Ganz™ (SG) pulmonary artery catheter (Edwards Lifesciences, Irvine, Calif) is placed via the right internal jugular vein.

A thin-walled (15-Fr or 17-Fr) Bio-Medicus™ cannula (Medtronic, Minneapolis, MN) is passed via the right internal jugular vein (double-puncture method with SG) into the distal superior vena cava. With the patient in a 30° right chest elevated position, he/she is prepared and draped sterilely. The right femoral artery is cannulated using either a 17 or 19-Fr Bio-Medicus™ cannula. For inferior vena caval drainage either 23 or 25-Fr RAP™ femoral venous cannula (Estech, San Ramon, CA) is passed over a guide-wire into the right atrium. Vacuum-assisted venous drainage is used in all of these operations.

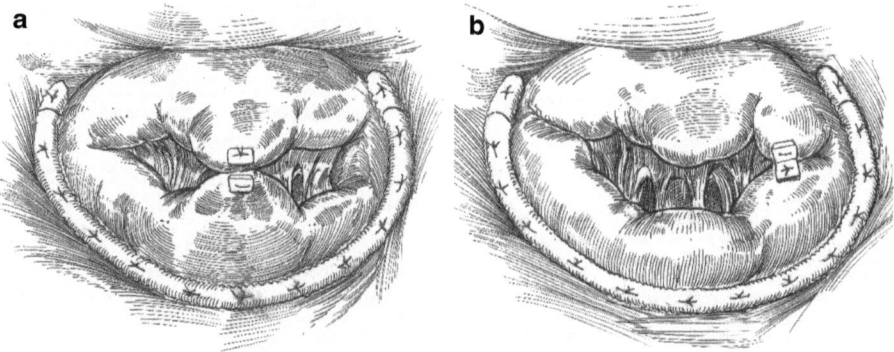

**Fig. 4.6** (**a**) Double orifice repair: The edge-to-edge technique, shown here, is used to repair large segments of redundant mitral leaflet. This is especially applicable to central mitral valve leaks. (**b**) Para-commissural repair: The edge-to-edge technique, shown here, is used to repair prolapsing valve regions that are either near or at the commissures (With permission from [9])

### 4.5.2  Aortic Occlusion and Myocardial Protection

We prefer the trans-thoracic aortic clamp method as it has been proven to be safe, reliable, economic, and simple to apply. For myocardial protection we use a systemic blood inflow temperature of 28 °C with cold antegrade crystalloid Bretschneider's HTK cardioplegia solution. When infusing cardioplegia, the dynamic retractor should be lowered to avoid aortic valvular incompetence.

Carbon dioxide is insufflated continuously through the right robotic arm side-port. Following the left atriotomy and mitral valve exposure, a weighted sucker is placed in the left superior pulmonary vein to remove remaining intra-atrial blood. After completing the repair and before atrial closure, this sucker is passed into the left ventricle as a vent. The left atrium is closed with a running 4-0 PTFE suture by the console surgeon. The heart is de-aired by inflow filling, while ventilating and applying suction to the aortic root vent. CPB weaning is by our standard protocol.

### 4.5.3  Edge-to-Edge Robotic Mitral Repair

As mentioned earlier, determination of precise regurgitant sites is important. At these leaks, the free edge of the diseased leaflet will be sutured to the corresponding opposing leaflet edge. For the central valve regurgitation, this technique produces a double valve orifice (Fig. 4.6a). Para-commissural repairs result in a single orifice but with a slightly reduced valve area (Fig. 4.6b). Multiple regurgitant jets in (Barlow's) bileaflet prolapse often can be corrected by suture approximation of the middle portions ($A_2$ to $P_2$) of the anterior and posterior leaflets. Alfieri and colleagues showed that EE repairs should be followed with a ring annuloplasty to provide the best long-term outcomes. We prefer not to use the EE technique when the annular size is small (<34 mm ring sizer) or with stiff leaflets, resulting from subvalvular fibrosis, as mitral stenosis can be created.

We perform either a "double orifice" or "para-commissural repair," depending on definition of the diseased leaflet segments. Using robotic Resano forceps, all prolapsing or flail leaflet segments are located. In the presence of mid-scallop ($P_2$) posterior leaflet prolapse or flail, the precise middle of anterior leaflet ($A_2$) is defined. Thereafter, we attach the dysfunctional segment to the opposite leaflet in the rough zone at the same geometric level first using a polyamide monofilament 4-0 Cardionyl™ "stay" suture (Peters Surgical, Paris, France). Beware that if the posterior and anterior leaflet portions are suture approximated off center or "skewed," the EE repair will not be successful. Chords that converge at leaflet edges from both papillary muscles denote the "anatomical middle" and are a guide for approximation.

We estimate the size of each residual orifice with a linear (mm) ruler and from the size of the instrument arms (12-mm in diameter). In sternotomy-based operations, we use Hagar dilators to estimate each orifice size. A post-repair total valve area of greater than 2.5 cm$^2$ is considered acceptable for "normal size" patients. At this time pressurized left ventricular saline filling helps determine the adequacy of the two orifices, leaflet coaptation symmetry, and valve competence.

After confirmation of leaflet symmetry, we use 4-0 PTFE sutures to complete the EE approximation (Fig. 4.7b). Material strength and low fracture rate with robotic instruments makes PTFE suture ideal for these mitral repairs. For the double orifice repair, deep running suture bites are taken along $A_2$ and $P_2$. We suggest deploying a "mattress" suture line first followed by an "over and over" second suture line. These sutures should be placed deep in the "rough zone" to reduce tissue redundancy. The length of suture line should be kept short (10–15 mm) to reduce the risk of valvular stenosis but provide a stable repair. Occasionally, we will use a small pledget to reinforce the repair.

An annuloplasty is performed in conjunction with all repairs to restore the native geometry, reduce the annular size, prevent further dilatation, and reinforce the repair. Moreover, reducing the anterior–posterior annular diameter increases the leaflet coaptation surface. In all of our robotic mitral valve repairs, we have used the Edwards Cosgrove Annuloplasty Band System™ (Edwards Lifesciences, Irvine Calif.), as the inter-trigonal distance is usually normal in degenerative mitral valves (Fig. 4.7c). As mentioned before, we select the annuloplasty band size based on our intra-operative echocardiographic data. We believe that a "trigone to trigone" posterior band provides optimal coaptation while preserving a "saddle-shaped" systolic configuration. Alfieri has shown the long-term results are inferior to repairs having a ring or band annuloplasty [8].

In most instances we have anchored the band using 2-0 Cardioflon™ braided suture (Peters Surgical, Paris, France) with intra-corporeal tying. We begin our suturing method at the right fibrous trigone with the first two sutures delivered backhand. The remaining sutures are placed forehand, continuing in a clockwise direction. Most recently we have used 2-0 Ticron™ braided sutures (Covidien, Mansfield, MA) with annuloplasty band suture fixation using the automated Cor-Knot ™ (LSI Solutions, Victor, NY) device (Fig. 4.8). After passing both 2-0 Ticron™ sutures through the band, they are brought through a wire loop. The loop is then withdrawn

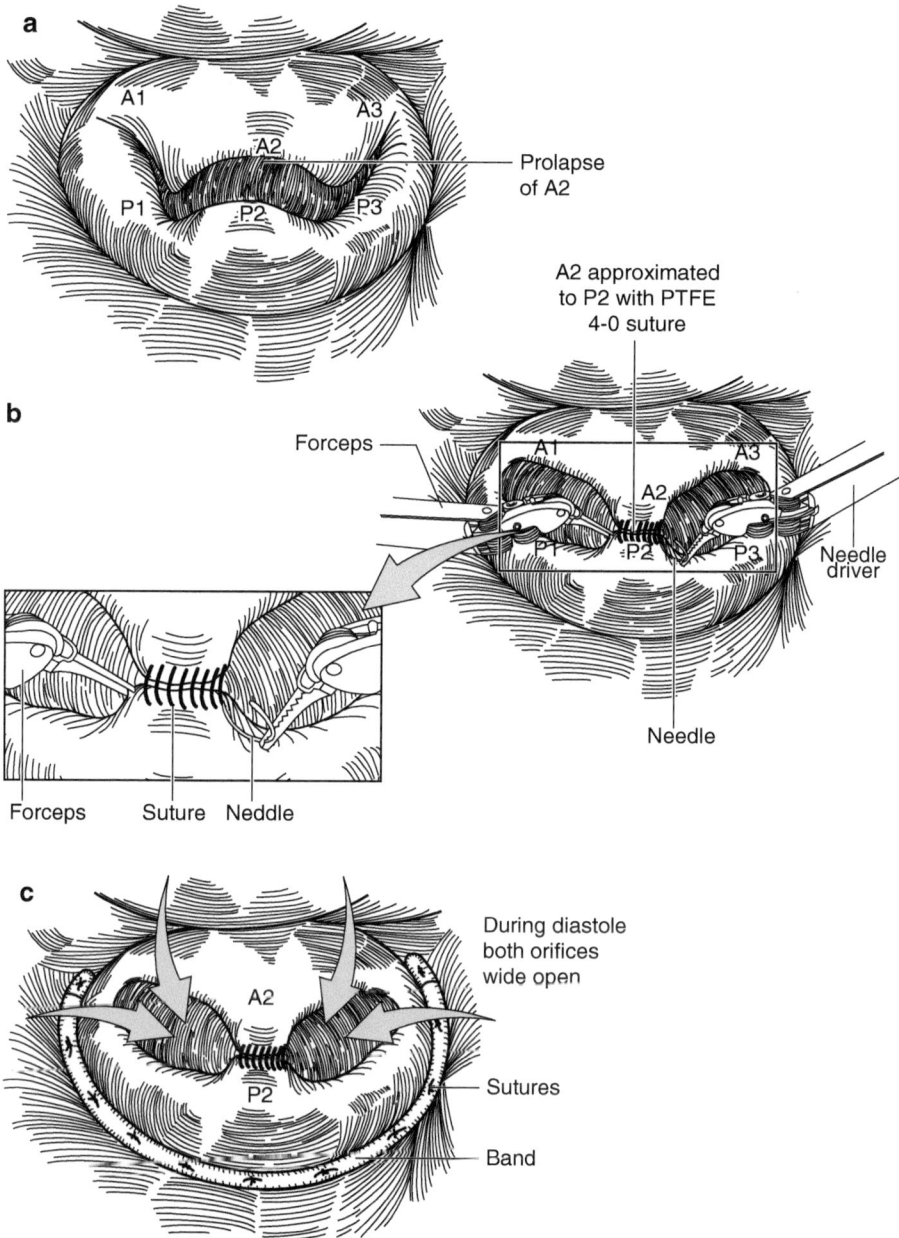

**Fig. 4.7** Robotic double orifice edge-to-edge repair. (**a**) This shows severe anterior leaflet pro-lapse mainly in the $A_2$ region as well as moderate $P_2$ prolapse. (**b**) Robotic Instruments are being shown approximating the large prolapsing $A_2$ to the posterior $P_2$ scallop using a two-later running 4-0 PTFE suture. (**c**) The double orifice repair is complete with the annuloplasty band implanted. Trans-mitral blood flow is shown through both orifices during diastole

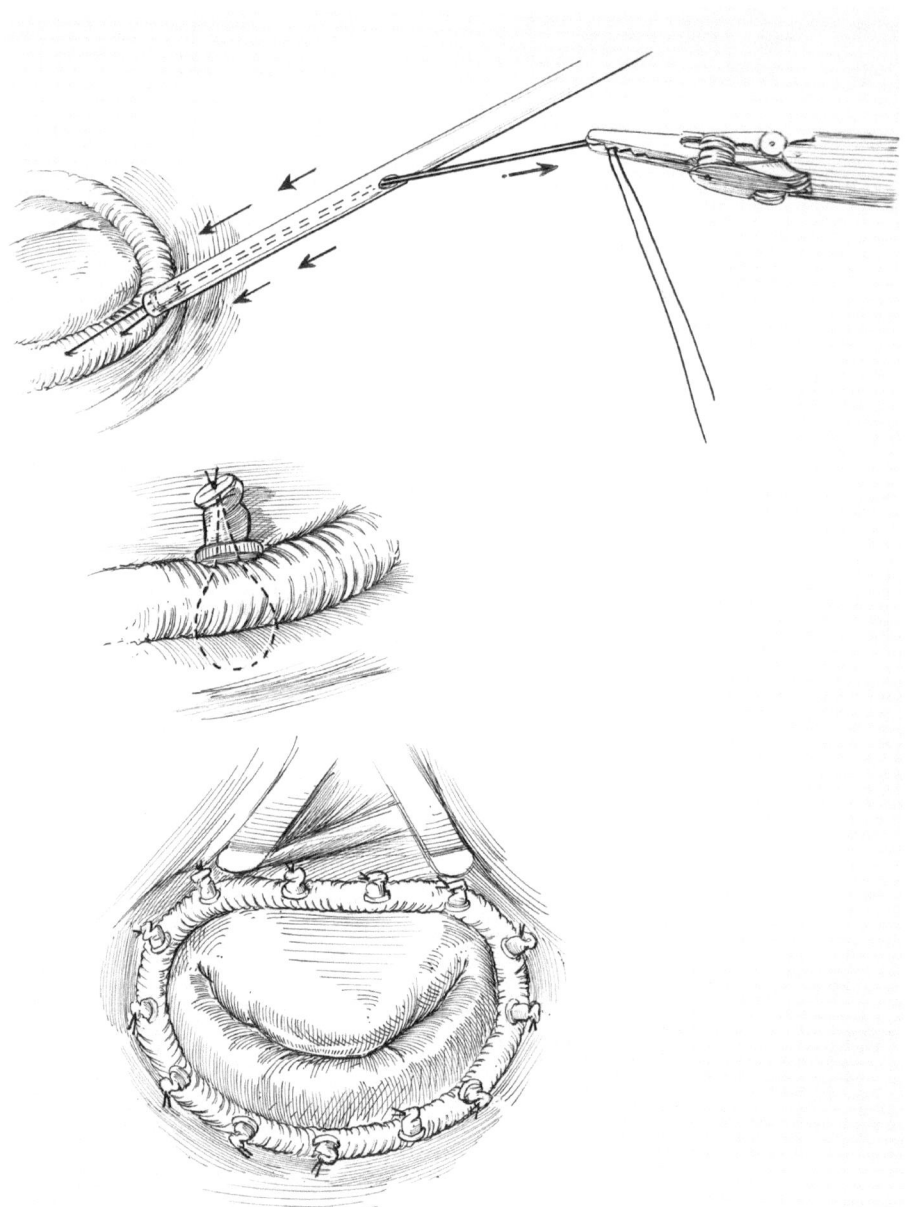

**Fig. 4.8** Core-Knot™ annuloplasty deployment: The Cor-Knot™ device facilitates annuloplasty band suturing. After 2-0 braded sutures are placed, the wire loop tip withdraws suture tails through the applier tip and a titanium "shim." The applier tip then is pressed against the band to tighten the suture. Thereafter, the applier is fired, crimping the metal shim on the suture and cutting it (With permission from [9])

through the applier (which brings both suture tails through a titanium shim). While simultaneously applying counter traction on the sutures, while firmly applying the shaft tip against the band, the device is fired securing and cutting the suture. We have found this method to be ideal as it saves operative time.

## 4.6    Outcomes

Since 2000 we have done over 920 robotic mitral repairs with 30 of them operated using the robotic edge-to-edge technique. Of these 12 had a concomitant cryomaze (Cox IV) procedure for atrial fibrillation. As mentioned above, most of the time we have reserved the EE for higher risk patients with either anterior and/or posterior leaflet prolapse. Also, in a few circumstances, it has been effective to correct a residual leak after a repair using another technique.

Of the series 25 patients were primary operations and five were reoperations. In six patients hypothermic ventricular fibrillation was used, and the remainder underwent aortic clamping with antegrade cold cardioplegia. There was one in-hospital death, and one patient had to be reoperated upon 5 months later for residual mitral stenosis. The mean patient age was 62 years and 83 % had severe mitral regurgitation. Of these 83 % had Carpentier type 2 insufficiency with 10 % having Type 1 and 7 % having Type 3 disease. Of this cohort 53 % had bileaflet prolapse. A band annuloplasty was added to the EE repair in 90 % of patients with an average band size of 34-mm. After the repair no patient had either a moderate or severe residual leak by trans-esophageal echocardiography. There were no infections, strokes, myocardial infarctions, or phrenic nerve injuries. One patient required a pacemaker before discharge. The hospital length of stay was 7.3 days with 46 % being discharged within 5 days of surgery.

### Conclusions

Although the edge-to edge technique has not been the mainstay of our mitral repair armamentarium, we have found it very effective in selected patients. The technique is applied easily to robotic technology. The superior instrument articulation and vision with robotics provide an optimal way to apply the EE through the least invasive incisions. Professor Alfieri proved the long-term efficacy of this method, and robotic cardiac surgeons should put the EE in their operative "toolbox" either as their primary repair choice or for selected patients.

## References

1. Nifong LW, Chu VF, Bailey BM, Maziarz DM, Sorrell VL, Holbert D, Chitwood Jr WR. Robotic mitral valve repair: experience with the da Vinci system. Ann Thorac Surg. 2003;75(2):438–42; discussion 443.
2. Nifong LW, Chitwood WR, Pappas PS, Smith CR, Argenziano M, Starnes VA, Shah PM. Robotic mitral valve surgery: a United States multicenter trial. J Thorac Cardiovasc Surg. 2005;129(6):1395–404.

3. Nifong LW, Rodruiguez E, Chitwood WR. 540 Consecutive robotic mitral valve repairs including concomitant atrial fibrillation cryoablation. Ann Thorac Surg. 2012;94:38–43.
4. Suri RM, Antiel RM, Burkhart HM, Huebner M, Li Z, Eton DT, Topilsky T, Sarano ME, Schaff HV. Quality of life after early mitral valve repair using conventional and robotic approaches. Ann Thorac Surg. 2012;93:761–9.
5. Mihaljevic T, Jarrett CM, Gillinov AM, Williams SJ, DeVilliers PA, Stewart WJ, Svensson LG, Sabik JF, Blackstone EH. Robotic repair of posterior mitral valve prolapse versus conventional approaches: potential realized. J Thorac Cardiovasc Surg. 2011;141:72–80.
6. Maisano F, Torracca L, Oppizzi M, Stefano PL, D'Addario G, La Canna G, Zogno M, Alfieri O. The edge-to-edge technique: a simplified method to correct mitral insufficiency. Eur J Cardiothorac Surg. 1998;13:240–6.
7. Alfieri O, Maisano F, De Bonis M, Stefano PL, Torracca L, Oppizzi M, La Canna G. The double-orifice technique in mitral valve repair: a simple solution for complex problems. J Thorac Cardiovasc Surg. 2001;122:674–81.
8. De Bonis M, Lapenna E, Lorusso R, Buzzati N, Gelsomino S, Taramasso M, Vizzardi E, Alfieri O. Very long-term results (up to 17 years) with the double-orifice mitral valve repair combined with ring annuloplasty for degenerative mitral regurgitation. J Thorac Cardiovasc Surg. 2012;144:1019–24.
9. Chitwood WR, editor. Atlas of robotic cardiac surgery. New York: Springer; 2014.

# Echocardiographic Assessment of a Double-Orifice Mitral Valve: Tips and Tricks

5

Giovanna Di Giannuario, Emanuela Alati,
and Giovanni La Canna

## 5.1 Introduction

The edge-to-edge (EE) technique is also called "double-orifice mitral valve repair" when the suture of the two leaflets' free edges is performed centrally, therefore creating a double-orifice mitral valve (MV) (Fig. 5.1).

The mitral valve apparatus is a complex entity consisting of the left atrium, leaflets, annulus, chordae tendineae, papillary muscles, and left ventricular wall (Fig. 5.2). Pathological changes occurring in any of these components may lead to mitral valve dysfunction [1, 2].

In western countries, the most common etiology of mitral valve pathology is the degenerative disease, affecting around 2 % of the population and including a wide spectrum of anatomical lesions, from fibroelastic deficiency to extensive myxomatous degeneration as in Barlow's disease (Fig. 5.3). The second main cause of mitral disease is functional mitral regurgitation (FMR), which is secondary to ischemic and dilated cardiomyopathy.

Mitral valve reconstruction is currently the standard treatment for degenerative disease, functional MR, and, if the anatomy is favorable, also for some cases of infective endocarditis and rheumatic disease (Table 5.1, [2–4]). Although several surgical techniques have been developed for mitral valve repair, in this chapter we will focus only on the echocardiographic tips and tricks to evaluate the double-orifice MV repair [7–13]. From this point of view, three main settings need to be considered:

G. Di Giannuario (✉) • E. Alati • G. La Canna
Department of Cardiac Surgery, IRCCS San Raffaele
University Hospital, Via Olgettina, 60, Milan 20100, Italy
e-mail: gdigiannuario@gmail.com

© Springer International Publishing Switzerland 2015
O. Alfieri et al. (eds.), *Edge-to-Edge Mitral Repair: From a Surgical to a Percutaneous Approach*, DOI 10.1007/978-3-319-19893-4_5

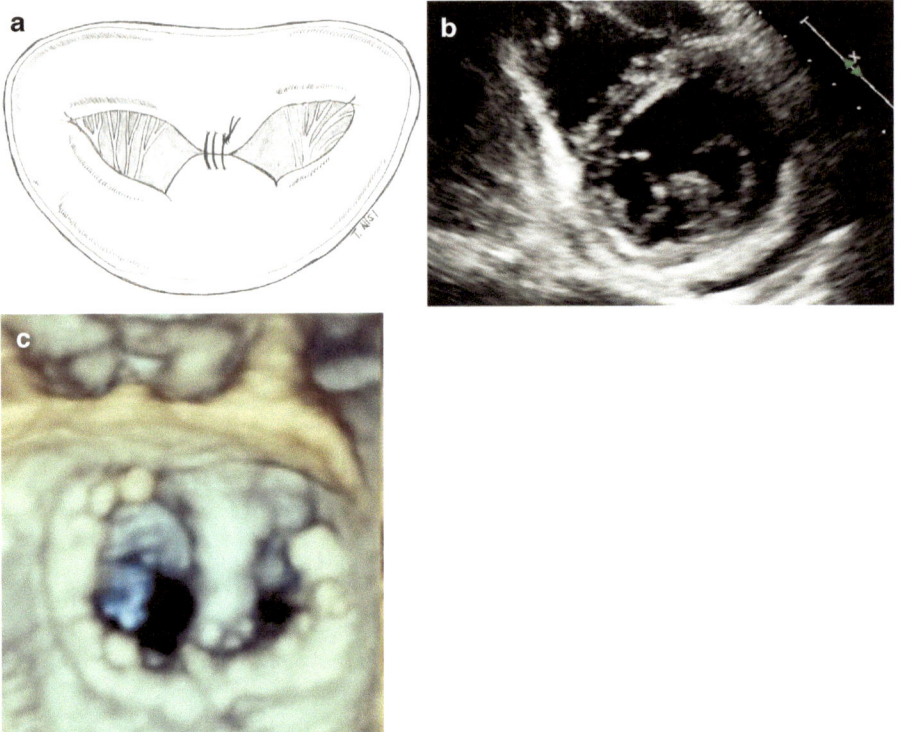

**Fig. 5.1** Anatomical characteristic of double-orifice technique compared a schematic representation (**a**) with 2D (**b**) and 3D zoom acquisition (**c**) echocardiography imaging

1. The preoperative setting, during which the severity of MR is assessed, the anatomical lesions are considered, and the possibility of performing an EE repair is evaluated.
2. The intraoperative setting, when the result of the EE repair is analyzed immediately after weaning from the extracorporeal circulation. In this phase, the anatomical and functional restoration of the repaired valve is studied, and in the case of residual MR, the underlying mechanism needs to be identified (SAM, residual prolapse, cleft, left ventricular dyssynchrony, ventricular dysfunction, etc.). In addition, the intraoperative echocardiography should define the possible impact on residual MR of the hemodynamic conditions, establish if a second pump run is needed, and exclude any iatrogenic mitral valve stenosis.
3. The postoperative setting, when the results of the surgical repair are assessed with the patient in stable hemodynamic conditions. This step includes also long-term follow-ups looking at any unfavorable outcome such as residual MR, hemolytic jet, endocarditis, SAM, and post-EE repair mitral valve stenosis.

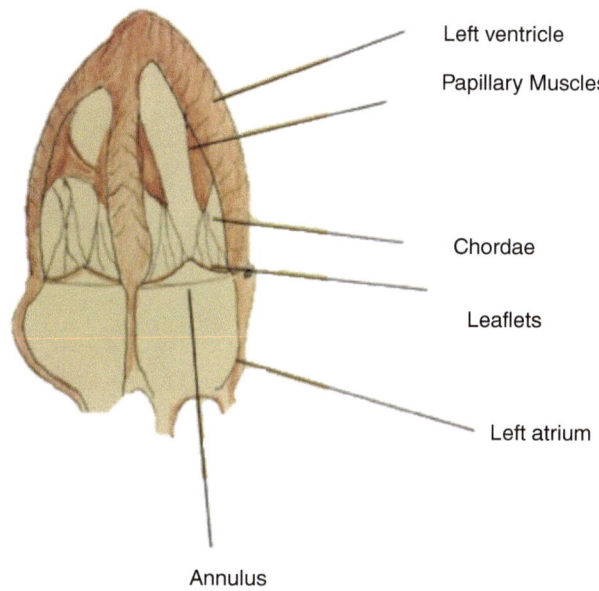

**Fig. 5.2** Mitral valve apparatus. Left ventricle, papillary muscles, chordae, leaflets, left atrium, annulus

Left ventricle

Papillary Muscles

Chordae

Leaflets

Left atrium

Annulus

**Table 5.1** Etiology of mitral valve disease suitable for MV repair

| |
| --- |
| Degenerative mitral disease |
|   Myxomatous disease |
|   Fibroelastic deficiency |
| Functional mitral disease |
|   Ischemic cardiomyopathy |
|   Dilated cardiomyopathy |
| Selected endocarditis disease |
| Selected rheumatic disease |

Moreover, in the current MitraClip era, we need also to consider the role of echocardiography in the selection of the patients, intraprocedural monitoring, and follow-up of the percutaneous double-orifice repair [14, 15].

### 5.1.1 Preoperative Setting: The Anatomical Characterization of the Lesion

#### 5.1.1.1 Tips and Tricks in Degenerative Mitral Valve Disease
In degenerative MV disease, the first step is to characterize the lesion anatomically, since there is a wide spectrum of lesions, ranging from fibroelastic deficiency to myxomatous disease and Barlow's syndrome. The identification of ruptured chordae ("flail") is also important (Fig. 5.3).

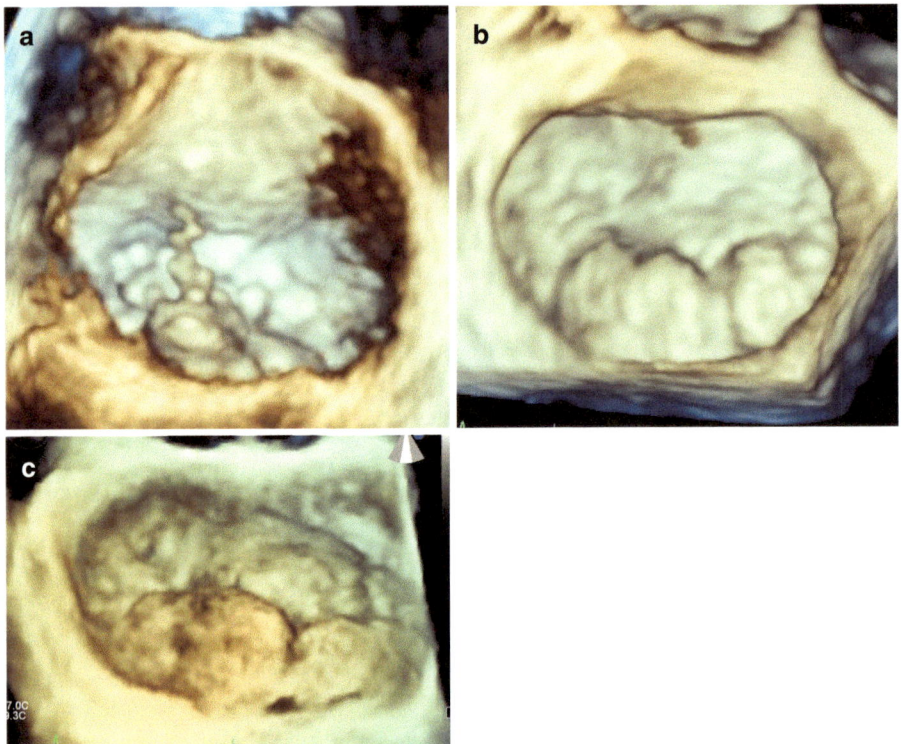

**Fig. 5.3** 3D zoom acquisition of different types of degenerative disease. Fibroelastic deficiency (**a**), myxomatous disease (**b**), Barlow's syndrome (**c**)

In this step, it is essential to establish whether the lesion is monoleaflet (anterior or posterior) or bileaflet and which segment or scallop of the leaflet is involved. In Carpentier's classification, the posterior leaflet is usually divided by two intraleaflet clefts into three scallops: P1 (anterolateral), P2 (central), and P3 (posteromedial). According to Duran's Classification, the scallop P2 may be divided into two sub-units: P2M1 (more anterolateral) and P2M2 (more posteromedial). On the other hand, in the anterior leaflet, there are normally no clefts and three segments (A1-A2-A3) can be identified, which are facing the corresponding P1, P2, and P3 scallops (Fig. 5.4). We can also identify two commissures: anterolateral (near the left appendage between P1 and A1) and posteromedial (between P3 and A3).

In case of bileaflet prolapse, it is important for the indication to the EE repair to describe if the lesions are facing or non-facing (Fig. 5.5).

This anatomical characterization helps to identify whether the mitral valve lesion is simple or complex and the likelihood of efficacy and durability of the repair (Table 5.3, [19]).

The preoperative anatomical characterization may be performed by transthoracic echocardiography and two-dimensional (2D) transesophageal echocardiography (TOE). The latter, through a multiplanar acquisition of different planes, is more

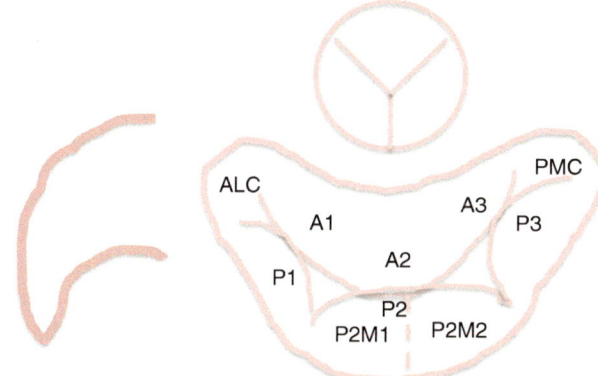

**Fig. 5.4** Carpentier's nomenclature of the mitral valve leaflet anatomy. The posterior leaflet is divided by two clefts in three scallops *P1* (anterolateral), *P2* (central), and *P3* (posteromedial). The anterior leaflet in a normal subject does not have any cleft. There are also two commissures: anterolateral (*ALC*) and posteromedial (*PMC*). According to Duran's classification, which follows the chordae insertion, the central scallop P2 is divided in two segments: *P2M1* (anterolateral) and *P2M2* (posteromedial)

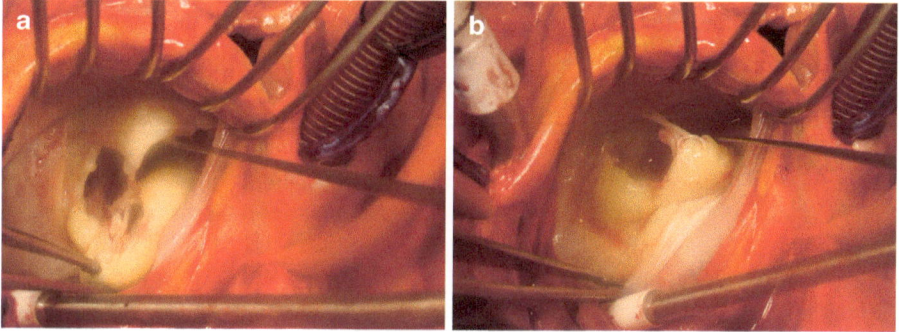

**Fig. 5.5** Intraoperative photos with "the surgical view" of a complex MV lesion, a bileaflet prolapse/flail of A2-P2 (facing segment). In the figure (**a**) it is showed a prolapse/flail of A2 and in the figure (**b**) it is showed a prolapse/flail of P2

detailed. Traditional ASE-SCA imaging planes and off-axis views may be used to explore the MV and reconstruct the three-dimensional image of the valve. The introduction of three-dimensional (3D) echocardiography in the clinical practice has simplified the examination of the mitral valve with the possibility of using 3D zoom, 3D full volume, and 3D color full volume acquisitions [20–22].

3D transesophageal echocardiography has changed the physician's ability to describe the mitral valve anatomy in the degenerative setting and has simplified the dialogue with the cardiac surgeon through 3D zoom acquisition with "surgical view" (Fig. 5.6).

3D transesophageal echocardiography is the most powerful, accurate, and specific technique to identify sites and types of prolapsing lesions. By using this method, we recently introduced a new classification of degenerative MV lesions, which distinguishes between dominant and secondary prolapses. In this study, the echocardiographic data were compared with the surgical findings, and per-patient analysis of real-time (RT) 3D-TOE identified the prolapse more accurately (92 %) than 2D-TOE (78 %), RT3D-transthoracic echocardiography (TTE, 80 %), and 2D-TTE (54 %). Indeed, the multiplanar reconstruction allows RT3D-TOE to differentiate between dominant ($\geq$5-mm displacement) and secondary (2 to <5-mm displacement) prolapses. By using the surgical findings as controls, the predicted value was 100 % for dominant lesions but only 34 % for secondary prolapses (Fig. 5.7) [5]. 3D zoom acquisition of the mitral valve allows to identify also the intraleaflet clefts and incisures (or pseudoclefts) that may normally be present in the posterior leaflet of a normal valve but may have a pathological role in degenerative MV disease since the diastasis of the clefts secondary to annular dilation may cause pathologic regurgitant jets [34].

There are several MV lesions for which the EE technique is appropriate: a segmental prolapse of the anterior leaflet in myxomatous disease or in fibroelastic deficiency, bileaflet prolapse of facing segments (i.e., A2-P2), and commissural lesions represent the most common indications (Table 5.2).

During the preoperative MV assessment, it is mandatory to establish if there is a calcification of the annulus (mild or severe, spot, or circumferential) and its extension to the leaflet's tissue, to the target lesion, or sometimes to the ventricular wall (Fig. 5.8). Indeed, the surgical experience with the EE technique indicates that the rate of recurrent MR at follow-up is high if the procedure is not associated with a ring annuloplasty for the presence of annular calcification [19].

Some anatomical conditions, such as small native valve area, intercommissural extension of the prolapsing lesion, intercommissural length of the surgical suture, and the use of a restrictive annuloplasty, represent important risk factors for the development of stenosis post-EE repair. Those variables need to be evaluated, and the surgeon using this technique should pay attention to them in order to leave an acceptable anatomical area (at least 2.5 cm$^2$ in normal size patients) (Chap. 9).

It is important to define the complexity of the MV lesions and the likelihood of a durable repair (Table 5.3). Finally, it is mandatory to assess the conditions predisposing to post-repair systolic anterior motion (SAM) of the anterior leaflet and dynamic obstruction of the left ventricle outflow tract (Table 5.4, [5–6, 16]). In some patients, the EE technique can be a simple solution to treat or prevent this complication [18].

In summary, in the preoperative setting, the echocardiographic assessment of degenerative MR includes the following tips and tricks:

- Tips
  - Type of degenerative MV disease (fibroelastic deficiency/myxomatous/ Barlow's syndrome)
  - Anatomical description of the degenerative disease (monoleaflet/bileaflet/ scallops involved)
  - Characterization of the lesion: simple/complex, facing/non-facing, dominant or secondary prolapse
  - Annular size and shape, presence, and extension of calcification

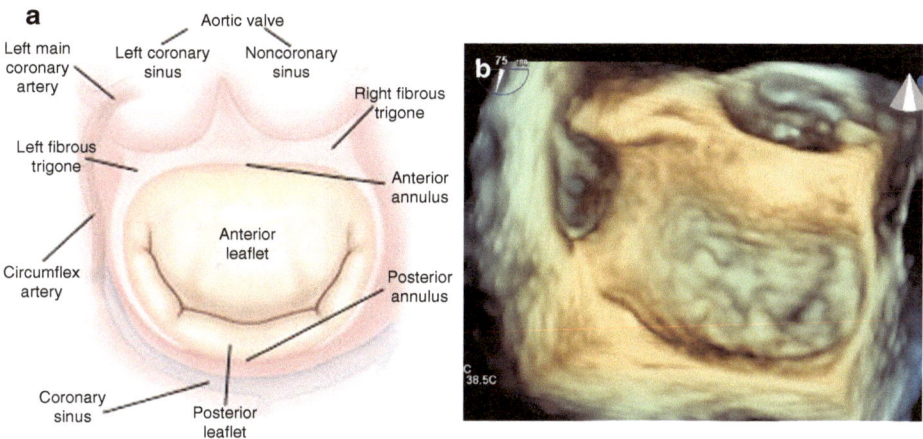

**Fig. 5.6** "The surgical view" of the mitral valve. (**a**) Schematic representation, (**b**) 3D zoom acquisition

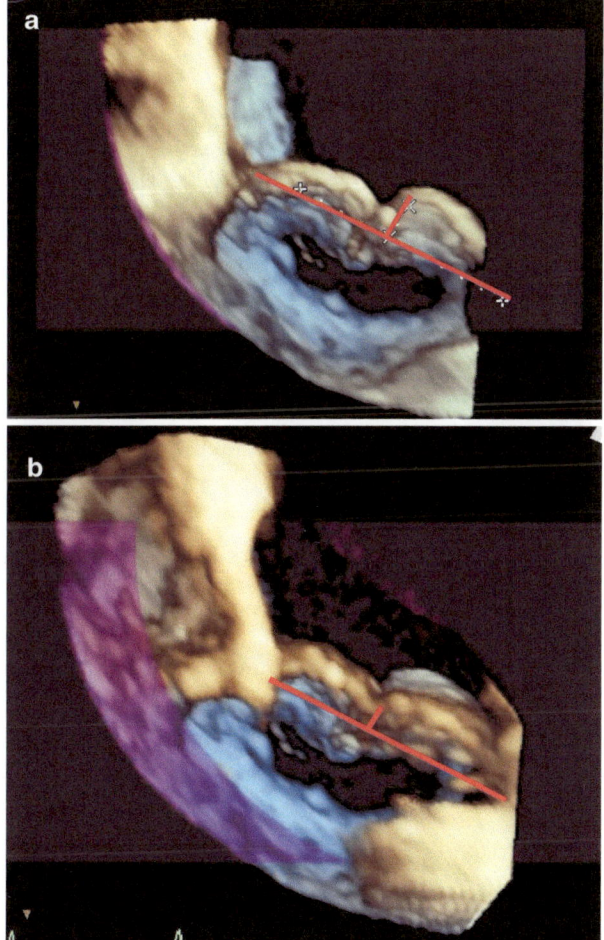

**Fig. 5.7** 3D zoom evaluation of degenerative mitral disease with evidence of dominant lesion (**a**) and secondary prolapse (**b**)

**Table 5.2** Anatomical indications and contraindications to the edge-to-edge repair

| Indications | Contraindications |
|---|---|
| Bileaflet prolapse (facing segments) | Intercommissural extension of prolapse lesion > 50 % <br> Calcification of the leaflets in target zone <br> Small valve area |
| Bileaflet prolapse (non-facing but adjacent segments: A2-P2M1 or A2-P2M2) | Intercommissural extension of prolapse lesion > 50 % <br> Calcification of the leaflets <br> Small valve area |
| Commissural prolapse | Calcification of the leaflets and the annulus |
| High risk of SAM | Small valve area |
| Residual MR after conventional repair (rescue EE) | Small valve area |
| Functional MR | Small valve area, extreme tethering |

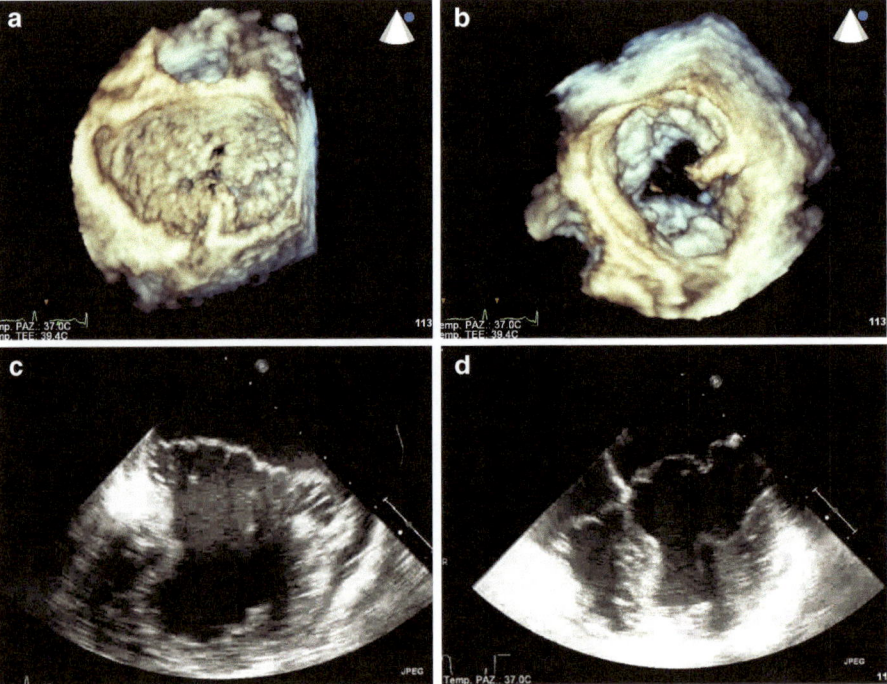

**Fig. 5.8** Annular calcification with extension to the mitral leaflet in a Barlow's syndrome. The calcification is evident only in the three-dimensional acquisitions (**a**) and (**b**) (3D TOE zoom). There is no evidence of calcification in the 2D TOE two-chamber and four-chamber midesopha-geal view (**c** and **d**)

**Table 5.3** Classification of simple and complex MV lesions and the related probability of successful and durable repair

|  | Simple lesion | Complex lesion | Lesion at high risk of unsuccessful repair |
|---|---|---|---|
| Type of lesion | Posterior leaflet prolapse/flail Annular dilation Leaflet perforation | Complex posterior leaflet lesions Anterior prolapse or flail Bileaflet prolapse or flail Combined lesions Deviant anatomy | Prolapse and extensive annular calcification Prolapse with hypoplasia of opposite leaflet Extreme fibroelastic deficiency Post-endocarditis leaflet damage Rheumatic disease |
| Probability of successful and durable repair | High | Depends on experience of the surgical team | Low |
| Needed expertise of the surgical team | Low | High | Very high |

Modified with permission from [19]

**Table 5.4** Risk factors for systolic anterior motion (SAM) and LVOT obstruction after MV repair

| Risk factors |  |
|---|---|
| Structural anomalies | Redundant anterior leaflet Redundant posterior leaflet Papillary muscle displacement Bulging septum Chordae anomaly (i.e., septum insertion) Small ventricle |
| Kinetic factors | Hyperdynamic left ventricle (localized or global) Catecholamine increase after CBP Metabolic or congenital disease |
| Geometric factors | Annular undersizing Anterior displacement of the mitral valve Low anterior-posterior leaflets' length ratio Reduced mitro-aortic angle Short distance between the mitral coaptation point and the septum |

- Risk factor of post-repair mitral stenosis
- Risk factors of systolic anterior motion
- Tricks
    - Use of 3D echocardiography zoom, 3D acquisition for anatomical characterization, and 3D cutting planes to assess the free margin of every scallop from anterolateral to posteromedial commissure (in order to identify dominant or secondary lesions)
    - 2D TOE short-axis transgastric view or 3D echo Q-lab (Philips Technology) to quantify the total orifice area of the native mitral valve and the intercommissural extension of the prolapsing lesion in order to avoid iatrogenic mitral stenosis

- Anatomical characterization of the leaflets, subvalvular apparatus, and papillary muscle position to prevent SAM
- Quantification of LVOT gradient (at rest, post-Valsalva maneuver, or under inotropic stimulation if necessary)
- Long-axis transgastric view to estimate the LVOT $V_{max}$ and maximum gradient in case of SAM
- Assessment of initial signs of LV deterioration in order to predict LV dysfunction post-EE repair

### 5.1.1.2 Tips and Tricks in Functional Mitral Regurgitation

The EE technique can be used to treat FMR secondary to ischemic or dilated cardiomyopathy (or to any other cause of left ventricular dilatation and dysfunction).

The mechanisms causing FMR are symmetrical or asymmetrical annular dilation, symmetrical or asymmetrical tethering of the leaflets, reduced LV systolic function, and LV remodeling.

There is strong evidence in the literature that FMR portends an adverse prognosis in patients with ischemic heart disease or dilated cardiomyopathy [23–32]. Hence, it is important to identify FMR, quantify its severity [14], and measure parameters which can have a role in the durability of the repair like coaptation depth, tenting area, posterior and anterior leaflet tethering angles, leaflet hypoplasia, annular or leaflet calcification, abnormal cleft diastasis, and native mitral valve orefice area (Figs. 5.9, 5.10, 5.11, and 5.12).

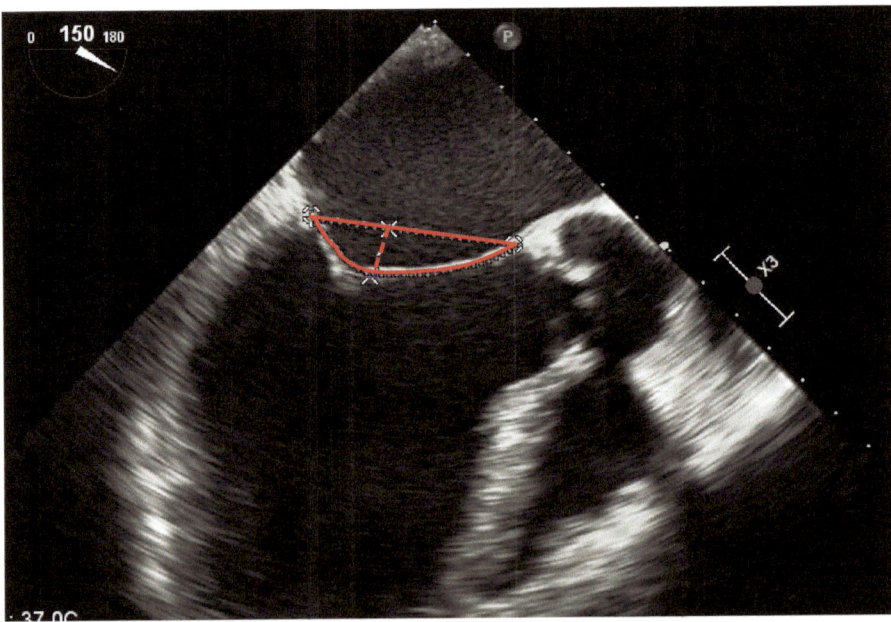

**Fig. 5.9** Functional MR with symmetric tethering and a coaptation depth <11 mm and tenting area <2 cm$^2$

**Fig. 5.10** Functional MR
with a posterior leaflet
angle<45°

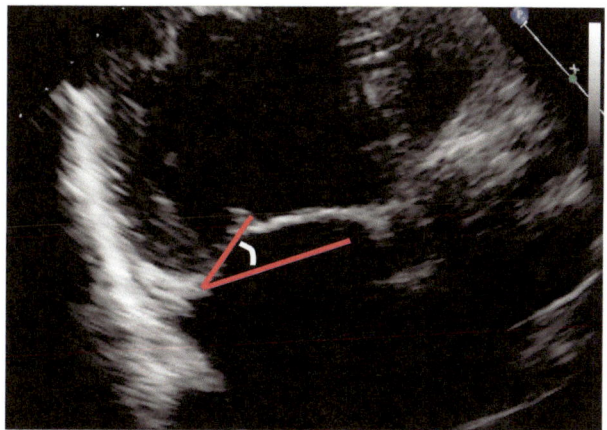

**Fig. 5.11** Functional MR
with an anterior leaflet
angle <25°

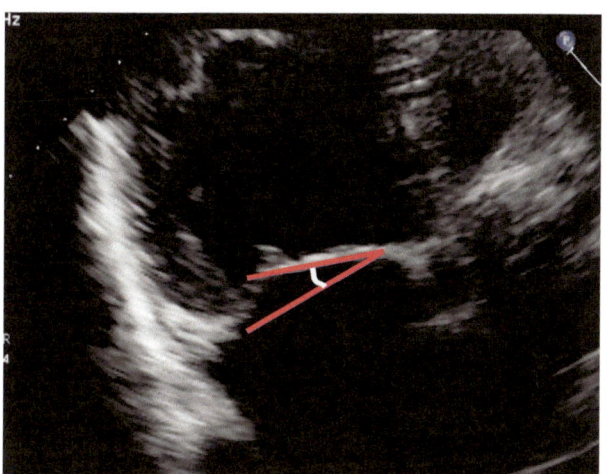

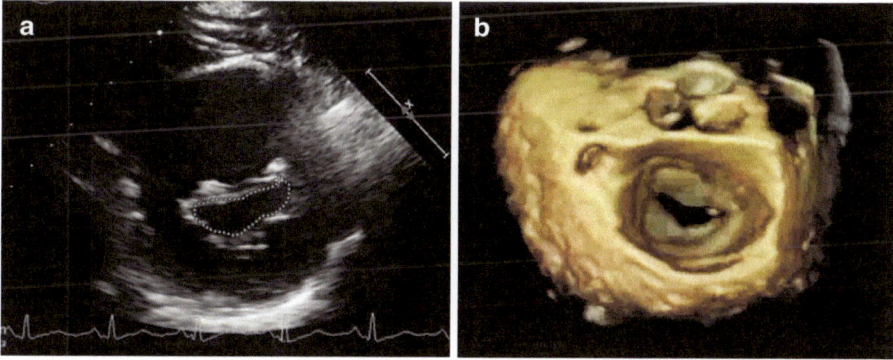

**Fig. 5.12** Planimetric evaluation of the native mitral valve area. A small area (<4 cm²) is a contra-indication to the EE technique for the high risk of post-repair mitral stenosis. 2D (**a**), 3D (**b**)

FMR is dynamic in nature and its echocardiographic quantitative evaluation may be affected by various factors: (1) loading conditions, (2) cardiac rhythm and arrhythmias, (3) dyssynchrony, (4) ischemia, and (5) possible negative pharmacological influence on the contraction forces [35].

The following echocardiographic parameters have been identified as predictors of a more durable surgical repair in FMR and should therefore be measured:

- Coaptation depth <11 mm
- Tenting area <2.5 cm$^2$
- Posterior leaflet tethering angle <45°
- Anterior leaflet tethering angle <25°
- Absence of severe hypoplasia of the leaflet
- Native mitral valve orefice area >4 cm$^2$

In the preoperative setting, the echocardiographic assessment of functional MR includes the following tips and tricks:

- Tips
  - Etiology of functional MR
  - Grading of fluctuating FMR
  - Anatomical characterization of the lesions
- Tricks
  - Echo stress dobutamine to assess the presence of left ventricular contractile reserve
  - Analysis of prognostic factors for a good repair
  - Evaluation of the factors influencing the "fluctuation" of FMR (also by using maneuvers able to modify these factors):
    - Loading conditions (preload and afterload)
    - Rhythm and arrhythmias
    - Dyssynchrony
    - Pharmacological therapy
    - Ischemia and viable myocardium (stress test)

## 5.1.2    The Intraoperative Transesophageal Echocardiography

After a double-orifice MV repair and at the end of the cardiopulmonary bypass, a transesophageal echocardiographic (TOE) evaluation of the final result is mandatory. The TOE echocardiography has to assess various factors:

1. Residual MR and the underlying mechanism (residual prolapse, SAM, cleft diastasis, suture dehiscence)
2. Double-orifice MV area (to exclude iatrogenic mitral stenosis)
3. Left ventricular dysfunction
4. Inferolateral ischemia due to circumflex artery iatrogenic occlusion
5. Paraprosthetic ring leak
6. Persistence of annular dilation

If a patient has an important contraindication to TOE (for instance, an esophageal diverticulum) or the TOE echocardiographic window is of poor quality, it is possible to investigate the double-orifice repair by trans-epicardial echocardiography, performed with the open chest in aseptic conditions in the operating room [20].

TOE examination is conducted according to the standard views identified by the main echocardiographic guidelines. It is possible to evaluate the morphology and function of the double-orifice valve by 2D TOE midesophageal (ME) four-chamber, long-axis (left ventricular outflow tract or three-chamber), two-chamber, intercommissural, and transgastric short- (useful to trace the double-orifice area) and long-axis views. The implementation of color Doppler allows the identification and quantification of any residual MR.

By using 3D echocardiography, the same information can be obtained in a more accurate and faster way with full volume rendering, color Doppler full volume, and 3D zoom acquisitions (Fig. 5.13, [21]).

Whenever a residual regurgitation is present, it is important to assess the localization (anterolateral or posteromedial, near the suture line, intraleaflet or interscallop, para-annular, commissural), the direction and the m-Mode time extention. In addition, a multiparametric quantification of MR has to be done.

Usually in the intercommissural and transgastric views, it is possible to establish whether the regurgitant jet is in the anterolateral or in the posteromedial orifice. The shape and direction of the jet are very important: usually a residual prolapse produces a jet directed towards the opposite side of the prolapsing segment, cleft diastasis or malapposition causes a centrally directed jet, and SAM is responsible for an eccentric jet directed towards the posteromedial atrial wall. In case of very eccentric jet, it is important to use off-axis views, in order to assess its real entity and direction (especially when the jet is directed towards the prosthetic ring and may induce severe hemolysis) (Fig. 5.14).

The transgastric long-axis view is important to identify any residual MR caused by left ventricular outflow tract obstruction and to assess LVOT gradient.

Continuous Doppler and pulsed-wave Doppler (PW) allow to calculate the max and mean transvalvular gradient and identify the presence of regurgitation.

In case of mild/moderate MR, it is important to assess the grade and position of the jet, the underlying mechanism of MR, and if a second pump run is needed.

### 5.1.2.1 The Impact of the Hemodynamic Conditions on the Intraoperative Echocardiographic EE Assessment

For the assessment of a residual regurgitation after EE repair in the intraoperative setting, it is very important to look at the hemodynamic conditions of the patient: volume load, systemic blood pressure, heart rate, heart rhythm, pacemaker stimulation, hematocrit and hemoglobin values, inotropic drugs, and mechanical ventilation (Fig. 5.15).

All these conditions can lead to under-/overestimation of the residual regurgitation. To assess the severity of residual MR, a multiparametric approach is usually required since many standard echocardiographic quantification methods are not helpful, being affected by different hemodynamic conditions. The site of origin of the regurgitant jet, the vena contracta, the left atrial extension of the color imaging, the m-Mode color time-related extension, the continuous color wave (CW), and the reverse flow in the upper pulmonary vein need to be assessed.

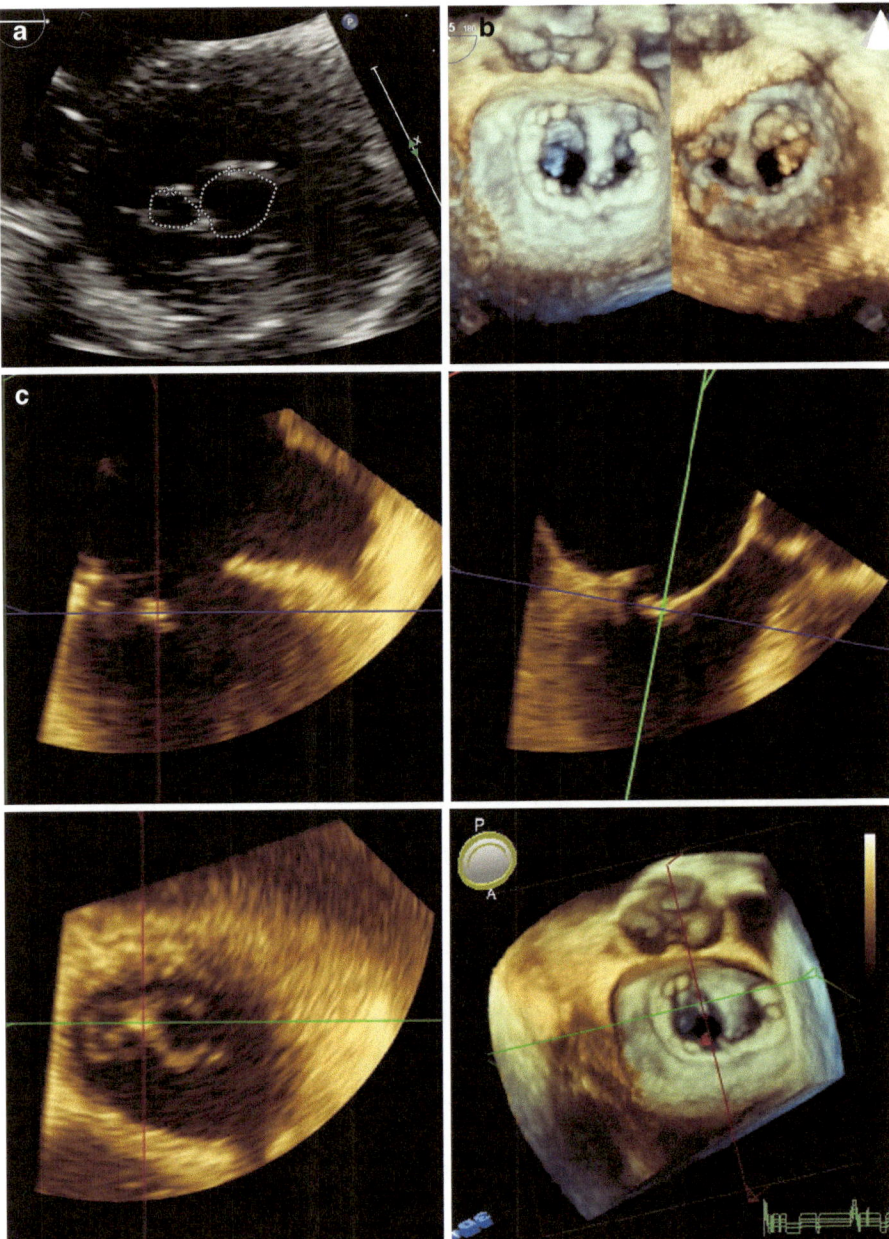

**Fig. 5.13** Double-orifice MV area. (**a**) 2D transgastric short-axis view, (**b**) 3D zoom acquisition (atrial and ventricular prospective), (**c**) Q-lab reconstruction for area quantification

After weaning from the cardiopulmonary bypass, it is important to wait for blood pressure and filling volume to return to physiologic conditions. Low systemic pressure and low filling volume may lead to underestimation, whereas high blood pressure, high filling volume, and low hematocrit or hemoglobin values may lead to overestimation of residual MR.

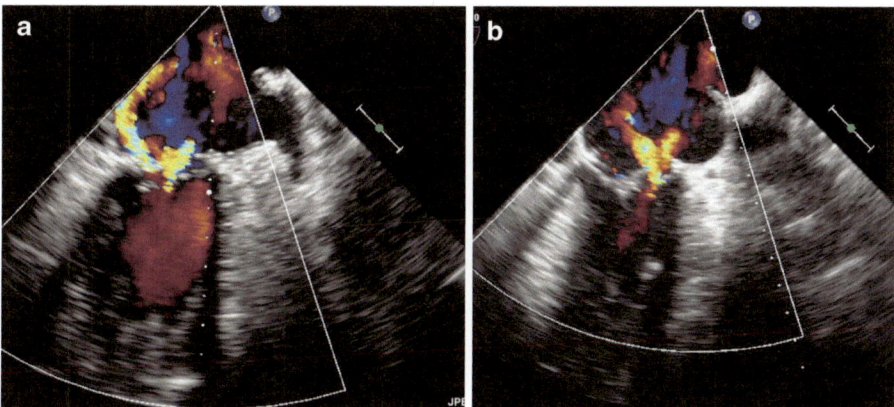

**Fig. 5.14** (**a, b**) 2D TOE imaging of post-repair eccentric jet, directed towards the posterior prosthetic annular ring and causing severe hemolytic anemia

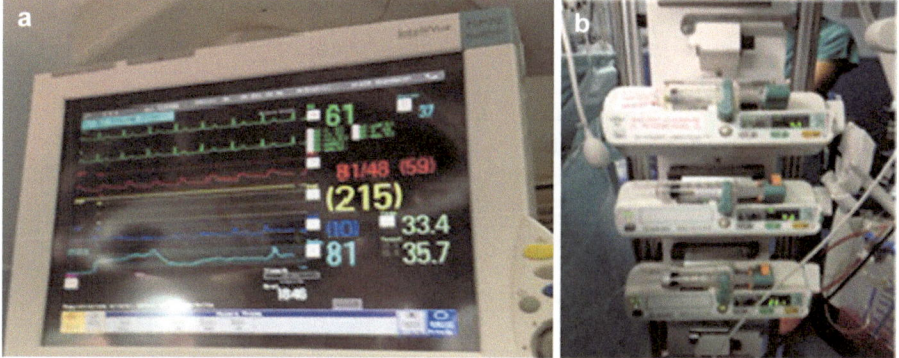

**Fig. 5.15** Intraoperative monitoring with hemodynamic parameters (**a**) and pumps for pharmacological infusions (**b**)

If some degree of residual MR is still present after optimal hemodynamic conditions have been achieved, several maneuvers will be necessary to assess the actual severity, the underlying mechanism, the possible reversibility, or the need for a second repair.

The main causes of residual regurgitation after EE repair are residual prolapse, cleft diastasis, SAM (asymmetrical, Fig. 5.16), suture dehiscence (Fig. 5.17), prosthetic ring dehiscence, and annular dilation.

Some maneuvers can be used to modify preload and afterload and establish if there is residual prolapse, malapposition, or SAM. Those maneuvers include partial ascending aorta cross-clamping, partial occlusion of the inferior vena cava, pharmacological manipulation, temporary interruption of the mechanical ventilation, volume administration, and changing of cardiac rhythm stimulation modality (optimizing AV pacing or resynchronization).

Modifying preload and afterload can influence the regurgitation gradient: an afterload increase usually induces an increase of the regurgitant gradient and a consequent reduction of prolapse or SAM-related regurgitation; a preload reduction

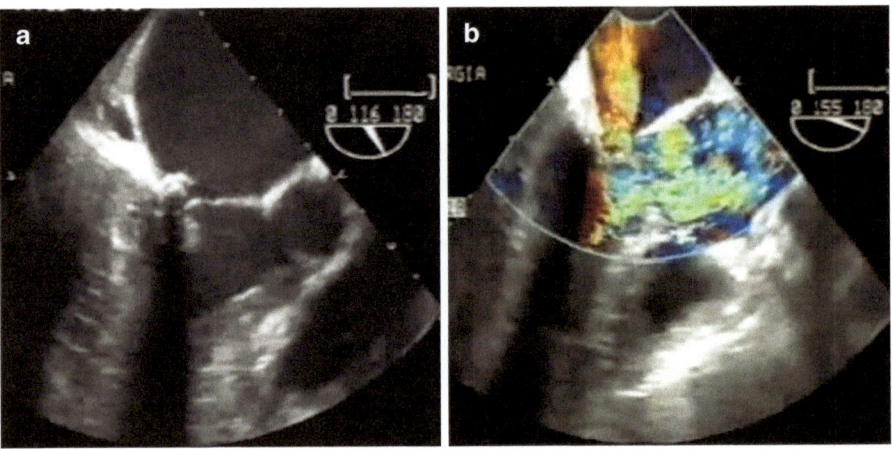

**Fig. 5.16** (**a**, **b**) Intraoperative transesophageal echocardiography showing systolic anterior motion (SAM) post-EE repair

decreases the regurgitant gradient and tends to increase prolapse or SAM-related regurgitation (Table 5.5).

If an intra-aortic balloon pump (IABP) is used in patients with FMR, this has to be switched off before the final evaluation of the results of EE repair.

In summary, in the intraoperative setting, the echocardiographic assessment of the EE repair includes the following tips and tricks:

- Tips
    - Multiplanar 2D TOE or 3D echo assessment of residual regurgitation and mechanism
        1. Apposition of the leaflets and morphology
        2. Color check of residual regurgitation
    - Transgastric view for the assessment of mitral stenosis (planimetric area)
    - Multiparametric evaluation of the grade of residual MR (convergent area, vena contracta, increase of left atrial pressure with systolic inversion in the two upper pulmonary veins)
- Tricks
    - Assess the final result in the best physiological conditions.
    - Use maneuvers to increase afterload (partial aortic clamping) or to decrease preload (partial occlusion of the inferior vena cava) to establish the real grade and mechanism of residual post-EE regurgitation.
    - 3D zoom acquisition for anatomical area.
    - Consider the potential masking effect of left ventricular ischemia or LV dyssynchrony (masking SAM or residual MR).
    - Transgastric long-axis view to differentiate SAM acceleration and its gradient from mitral valve regurgitation.
    - Check for pharmacological masking of SAM (noradrenalin, beta-blockers).
    - In case of FMR with severe LV dysfunction, evaluate the final result of the EE repair with IABP in switch-off mode.

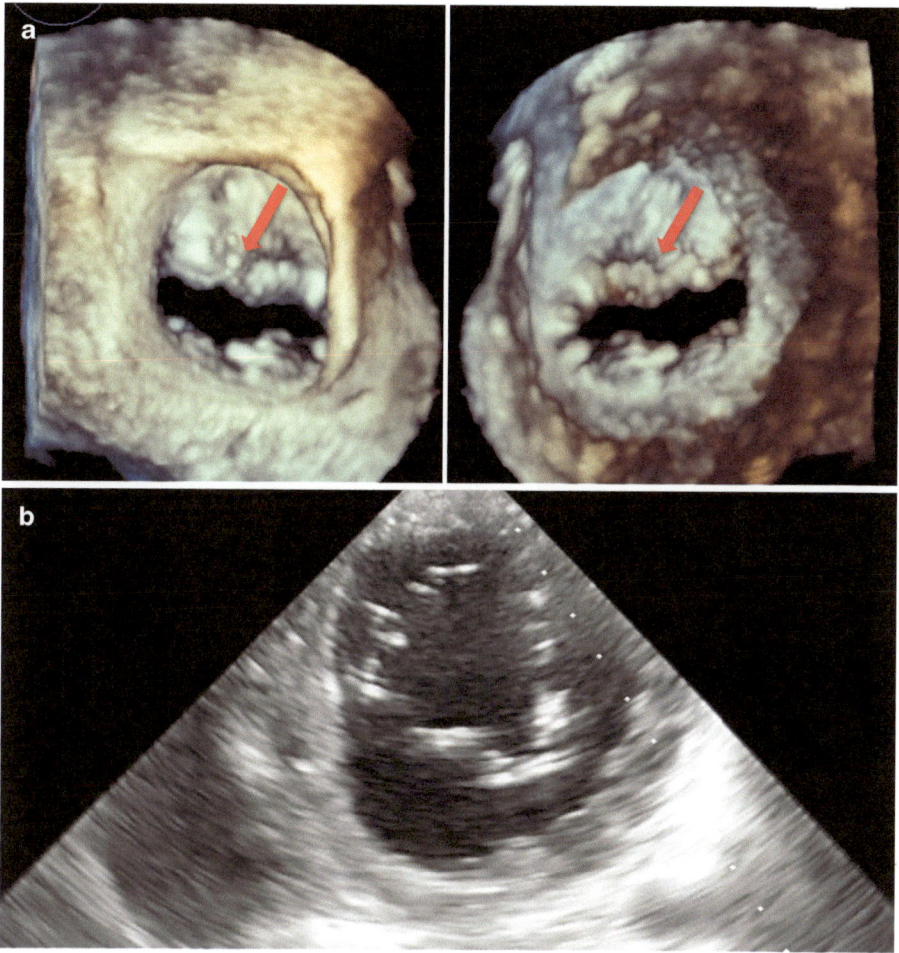

**Fig. 5.17**  3D (**a**) and 2D (**b**) TOE imaging of suture dehiscence after EE mitral valve repair

Stop the mechanical ventilation (which reduces the preload in the first phase).
- Be aware of the effect of pharmacologically induced hypotension (protamine can reduce preload and increase SAM and residual prolapse).
- The left ventricular vent may simulate mitral regurgitation and sometimes its shadow can mask MR.

### 5.1.3   The Postoperative Setting: Early and Late Follow-Up After EE Repair

In the early postoperative days, patients may usually be in a hyperdynamic state due to anemia, fever, or pain, and the transthoracic echocardiography examination can be of poor quality due to the reduced mobility of the patient and the high thoracic impedance. However, TTE remains important in looking for MR, iatrogenic stenosis, left ventricular dimensions and function, and pericardial effusion.

**Table 5.5** How the modification of preload and afterload can induce modifications in the grade of MR (from [20])

| Maneuver | Effect | Regurgitation gradient | Mechanism | | |
|---|---|---|---|---|---|
| | | | Prolapse | SAM | Retraction |
| Mechanical Load manipulation | | | | | |
| Partial Aortic clamping | ↑ Increase postload | ↑ Increase | ↓ Reduction | ↓ Reduction | ↑ Increase |
| Occlusion inferior vena cava | ↓ Reduction preload | ↓ Reduction | ↑ Increase | ↑ Increase | Not determined |
| Mechanical ventilation (first phase) | ↓ Reduction preload | ↓ Reduction | ↑ Increase | ↑ Increase | Not determined |
| Pharmacological manipulation | ↑ Increase postload | ↑Increase | ↓ Reduction | ↓ Reduction | Not determined |
| Volume expansion | ↑ Increase preload | ↑ Increase | ↓ Reduction | ↓ Reduction | ↑ Increase |
| Pacing AV delay Dyssynchrony | | ↑ Increase of diastolic gradient | ≠ No change Not determined | ≠No change Not determined | ↑ Increase ↓ Reduction |

In particular, at this stage, transthoracic echocardiography has to evaluate any residual regurgitation, its grade, the underlying mechanism (residual prolapse, SAM, cleft, endocarditis), and its potential evolution.

If the patient is symptomatic and has residual MR, a second-level examination (TOE or exercise stress echocardiography) is necessary to decide whether a reintervention is required.

In asymptomatic patients with recurrent significant MR, it is important to establish the hemodynamic impact of MR on the left ventricle and on the systolic pulmonary artery pressure. For this purpose, the patient has to be followed with repeated transthoracic examinations and exercise stress echocardiography. If during exercise echocardiography there is maladaptation, characterized by increased systolic pulmonary pressure (not due to an increase of systemic blood pressure) and exercise-induced left ventricular dysfunction, then reoperation will probably be necessary.

In our experience, we have also seen a few cases of SAM-related MR at midterm follow-up. In those patients, the rest echocardiographic examination is usually normal and only during exercise echocardiography SAM and MR can be induced and exertional dyspnea develops.

At long-term follow-up, if a repair failure occurs, transesophageal examination (2D or 3D) is essential to identify the mechanisms of this event (residual prolapse, cleft, suture dehiscence, new chordal rupture, endocarditis), the site of the regurgitation (posteromedial or anterolateral orifice), and whether it is commissural or near the suture line in order to decide between a possible second repair and a prosthetic replacement.

In summary, echocardiographic tips and tricks in the early and late postoperative stage after EE repair are:

- Tips
  - Residual regurgitation post-EE repair, grading, localization, mechanisms (SAM, cleft, endocarditis, suture dehiscence).
  - Assess post-EE repair mitral stenosis.
- Tricks
  - Utility of exercise test in asymptomatic patients with residual regurgitation.
  - Exercise test to investigate symptomatic patient for exercise dyspnea and normal rest echocardiographic findings.
  - 2D short-axis transgastric view TOE for the estimation of the mitral total orifice area (the sum of the two orifices) or 3D echo Q-lab quantification (Fig. 5.13).
  - 2D long-axis transgastric view TOE for the identification and quantification of LVOT gradient.
  - Check for eccentric intraleaflet or paraprosthetic ring jet that can cause hemolytic anemia (Fig. 5.14).

### 5.1.3.1 The Echocardiography in the Percutaneous Double-Orifice Repair with MitraClip System

In the last years, the percutaneous EE MitraClip system (Abbot Vascular) has been more extensively applied in high-risk patients [14, 15]. Selecting the suitable patients for the percutaneous EE is important. The EVEREST criteria have been widely used for this purpose. In our institution, in the degenerative setting, we distinguish between "simple lesion" (mainly P2 prolapse/flail) and "complex lesion" (commissural prolapse/flail, flail width >15 mm, bileaflet non-facing lesions). It is also important to identify any annular calcification and its extension to the leaflet tissue, cleft diastasis, and leaflet hypoplasia.

Similarly, in functional MR, we distinguish simple lesion (characterized by central jet), complex lesion, suboptimal lesion, and unfavorable lesion according to our clinical experience.

During the percutaneous procedure, the 2D and 3D transesophageal echocardiography is essential to guide: the transseptal puncture of the interatrial septum, the positioning of the delivery catheter, the orientation and positioning of the clip and to assess the final result of the procedure. Finally, echocardiography is needed to assess the early and long-term results.

Our echocardiographic tips and tricks in percutaneous EE repair can be summarized as follows:

- Tips
  - Identify the type of lesion and assess the feasibility of the procedure.
  - Assess calcification of the target lesion, cleft diastasis, leaflet hypoplasia, and loss of coaptation.
- Tricks
  - Use 2D and 3D TOE for a more accurate and specific evaluation of the anatomical lesion.

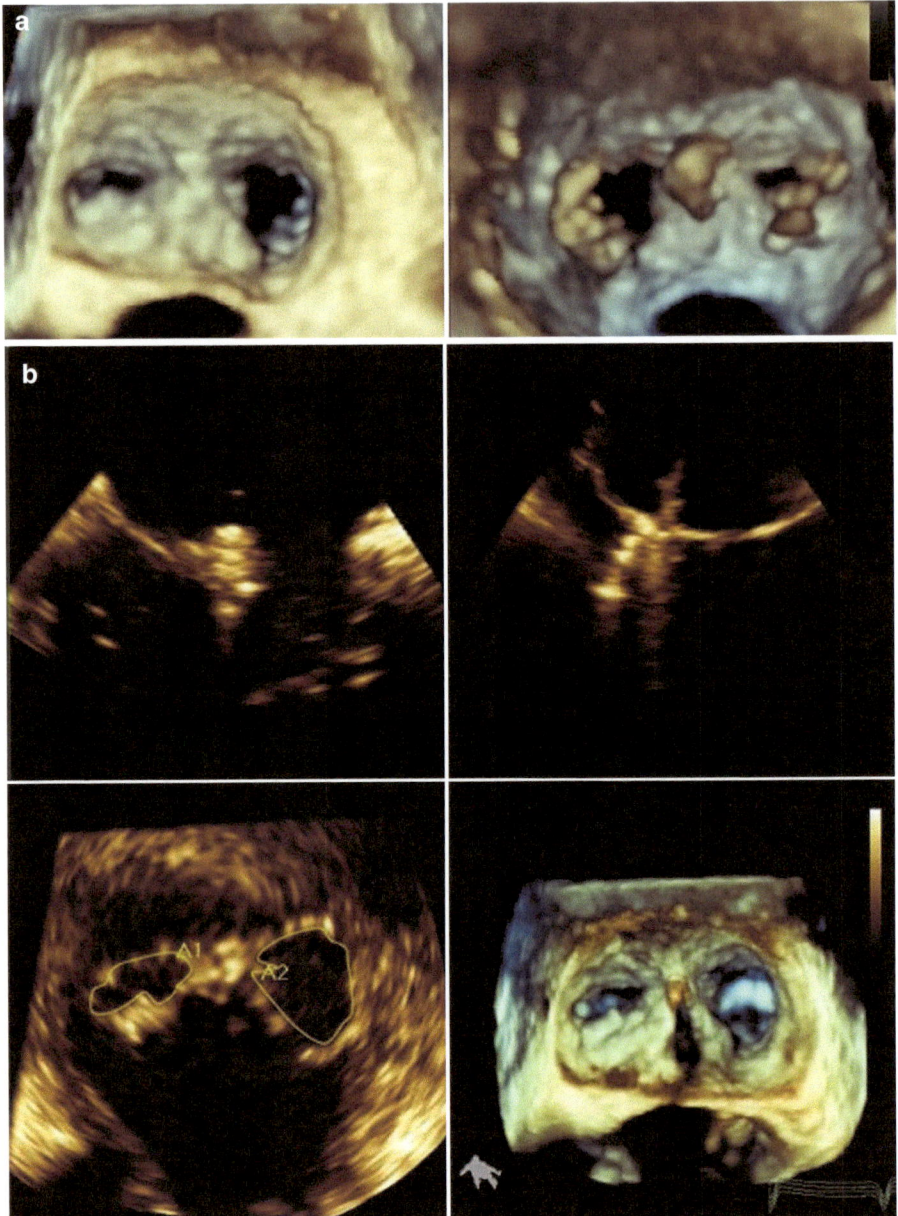

**Fig. 5.18** Double-orifice MitraClip implanatation. 3D zoom acquisition from atrial and ventricular views (**a**) and 3D analysis and reconstruction for the double-orifice area quantification (**b**)

- Use maneuvers that modify the loading condition for the assessment of residual regurgitation.
- Transgastric 2D/3D TOE zoom acquisition for post-repair double-orifice area (Fig. 5.18).

**Conclusion**

The echocardiographic assessment of a double-orifice mitral valve requires skill, knowledge, and experience. In the preoperative setting, 2D or 3D TOE examination can help to understand the mechanism of mitral disease and predict the feasibility and durability of the EE repair. In the intraoperative setting, if residual MR is present, it is very important to understand the mechanism of the residual regurgitation also by using specific maneuvers which can help to better define the real meaning of the residual MR. Different intraoperative conditions can modify or mask the real mechanisms and grade of the residual regurgitation, and our tips and tricks can help to avoid possible misdiagnosis. The evolution of 3D echocardiographic technique has improved our ability to detect anatomical lesions and assess the mechanisms of EE failure. Finally, early and late echocardiographic follow-ups of patients subjected to EE repair are an important instrument of clinical care.

# References

1. Devereux RB, Perloff JK, Reichek N, Josephson ME. Mitral valve prolapse. Circulation. 1976;54(1):3–14.
2. Messika-Zeitoun D, Topilsky Y, Enriquez-Sarano M. The role of echocardiography in the management of patients with myxomatous disease. Cardiol Clin. 2013;31(2):217–29.
3. De Kerchove L, Vanoverschelde JL, Poncelet A, Glineur D, Rubay J, Zech F, Noirhomme P, El Khoury G. Reconstructive surgery in active mitral valve endocarditis: feasibility, safety and durability. Eur J Cardiothorac Surg. 2007;31(4):592–9.
4. Filsoufi F, Carpentier A. Principles of reconstructive surgery in degenerative mitral valve disease. Semin Thorac Cardiovasc Surg. 2007;19(2):103–10.
5. Ibrahim M, Rao C, Ashrafian H, Chaudhry U, Darzi A, Athanasiou T. Modern management of systolic anterior motion of the mitral valve. Eur J Cardiothorac Surg. 2012;41(6):1260–70.
6. Sherrid MV, Gunsburg DZ, Moldenhauer S, Pearle G. Systolic anterior motion begins at low left ventricular outflow tract velocity in obstructive hypertrophic cardiomyopathy. J Am Coll Cardiol. 2000;36(4):1344–54.
7. Privitera S, Butany J, Cusimano RJ, Silversides C, Ross H, Leask R. Images in cardiovascular medicine. Alfieri mitral valve repair: clinical outcome and pathology. Circulation. 2002; 106(21):e173 4.
8. Alfieri O, Maisano F, De Bonis M, Stefano PL, Torracca L, Oppizzi M, La Canna G. The double-orifice technique in mitral valve repair: a simple solution for complex problems. J Thorac Cardiovasc Surg. 2001;122(4):674–81.
9. Yun KL, Miller DC. Mitral valve repair versus replacement. Cardiol Clin. 1991;9:315–27.
10. Gillinov AM, Cosgrove DM, Blackstone EH, Diaz R, Arnold JH, Lytle BW, et al. Durability of mitral valve repair for degenerative disease. J Thorac Cardiovasc Surg. 1998;116:734–43.
11. Carpentier A. Cardiac valve surgery – the "French correction". J Thorac Cardiovasc Surg. 1983;86(3):323–37.
12. Bhudia SK, McCarthy PM, Smedira NG, Lam BK, Rajeswaran J, Blac EH. Edge-to-edge (Alfieri) mitral repair: results in diverse clinical settings. Ann Thorac Surg. 2004;77(5): 1598–606.
13. Torracca L, Lapenna E, De Bonis M, Kassem S, La Canna G, Crescenzi G, Castiglioni A, Grimaldi A, Alfieri O. Minimally invasive mitral valve repair as a routine approach in selected patients. J Cardiovasc Med. 2006;7(1):57–60.
14. Feldman SK, Rinaldi M, Fail P, Hermiller J, Smalling R, Whitlow PL, et al. Percutaneous mitral repair with the MitraClip system: safety and midterm durability in the initial EVEREST (Endovascular Valve Edge-to-Edge REpair Study) cohort. J Am Coll Cardiol. 2009;54(8): 686–94.

15. Tamburino C, Ussia GP, Maisano F, Capodanno D, La Canna G, Scandura S, Colombo A, Giacomini A, Michev I, Mangiafico S, Cammalleri V, Barbanti M, Alfieri O. Percutaneous mitral valve repair with the MitraClip system: acute results from a real world setting. Eur Heart J. 2010;31(11):1382–9.
16. Mascagni R, Al Attar N, Lamarra M, Calvi S, Tripodi A, Mebazaa A, Lessana A. Edge-to-edge technique to treat post-mitral valve repair systolic anterior motion and left ventricular outflow tract obstruction. Ann Thorac Surg. 2005;79(2):471–3.
17. Hilberath JN, Eltzschig HK, Shernan SK, Worthington AH, Aranki SF, Nowak-Machen M. Intraoperative evaluation of transmitral pressure gradients after edge-to-edge mitral valve repair. PLoS One. 2013;8(9):e73617.
18. De Bonis M, Lapenna E, Buzzatti N, Taramasso M, Calabrese MC, Nisi T, Pappalardo F, Alfieri O. Can the edge-to-edge technique provide durable results when used to rescue patients with suboptimal conventional mitral repair? Eur J Cardiothorac Surg. 2013;43(6):e173–9.
19. De Bonis M, Maisano F, La Canna G, Alfieri O. Treatment and management of mitral regurgitation. Nat Rev Cardiol. 2011;9(3):133–46.
20. Nicolosi GL, Antonini-Canterin F, Pavan D, Piazza R. Manuale di Ecocardiografia Clinica. Padova: Piccin; 2008.
21. Savage RM, Aronson S, Shernan SK. Intraoperative transesophageal echocardiography. Philadelphia: Lippincott Williams and Wilkins; 2007.
22. Feigenbaum H, Armstrong WF, Ryan T. Feigenbaum's echocardiography. 6th ed. Philadelphia: Lippincott Williams and Wilkins; 2004.
23. Levine RA, Schwammenthal E. Ischemic mitral regurgitation on the threshold of a solution: from paradoxes to unifying concepts. Circulation. 2005;112:745–58.
24. Kwan J, Shiota T, Agler DA. Geometric differences of the mitral apparatus between ischemic and dilated cardiomyopathy with significant mitral regurgitation. Circulation. 2003;107:1135–40.
25. He S, Fontaine AA, Schwammenthal E, Yoganathan AP, Levine RA. Integrated mechanism for functional mitral regurgitation: leaflet restriction versus coapting force: in vitro studies. Circulation. 1997;96:1826–34.
26. Otsuji Y, Handschumacher MD, Schwammenthal E. Insights from three-dimensional echocardiography into the mechanism of functional mitral regurgitation: direct in vivo demonstration of altered leaflet tethering geometry. Circulation. 1997;96:1999–2008.
27. Kaul S, Pearlman JD, Touchstone DA, Esquival L. Prevalence and mechanisms of mitral regurgitation in the absence of intrinsic abnormalities of the mitral leaflets. Am Heart J. 1989;118:763–72.
28. Kono T, Sabbah HN, Rosman H, Alam M, Jafri S, Goldstein S. Left ventricular shape is the primary determinant of functional mitral regurgitation in heart failure. J Am Coll Cardiol. 1992;20:1594–8.
29. Lamas GA, Mitchell GF, Flaker GC. Clinical significance of mitral regurgitation after acute myocardial infarction: Survival and Ventricular Enlargement Investigators. Circulation. 1997;96:827–33.
30. Grigioni F, Enriquez-Sarano M, Zehr KJ, Bailey KR, Tajik AJ. Ischemic mitral regurgitation: long-term outcome and prognostic implications with quantitative Doppler assessment. Circulation. 2001;103:1759–64.
31. Trichon BH, Felker GM, Shaw LK, Cabell CH, O'Connor CM. Relation of frequency and severity of mitral regurgitation to survival among patients with left ventricular systolic dysfunction and heart failure. Am J Cardiol. 2003;91:538–43.
32. Deja MA, Grayburn PA, Sun B. Influence of mitral regurgitation on survival in the surgical treatment for ischemic heart failure trial. Circulation. 2012;125:2639–48.
33. Grayburn PA, Weissman NJ, Zamorano JL. Quantitation of mitral regurgitation. Circulation. 2012;126:2005–17.
34. La Canna G, Arendar I, Maisano F, Monaco F, Collu E, Benussi S, De Bonis M, Castiglioni A, Alfieri O. Real-time three-dimensional transesophageal echocardiography for assessment of mitral valve functional anatomy in patients with prolapse-related regurgitation. Am J Cardiol. 2011;107(9):1365–74.
35. Lancellotti P, Fattouch K, La Canna G. Therapeutic decision-making for patients with fluctuating mitral regurgitation. Nat Rev Cardiol. 2015;12(4):212–9.

# The Early Phase of Clinical Application: Lessons Learned

6

## Roberto Lorusso, Enrico Vizzardi, and Sandro Gelsomino

The experience of mitral valve repair (MVR) in the presence of anterior or bileaflet involvement has been not as satisfactory as the results of valve reconstruction for isolated posterior leaflet dysfunction [1–4]. Indeed, whereas quadrangular resection or other reparative techniques have been widely applied with remarkable long-lasting effects [5], mitral valve insufficiency (MVI) caused by mechanisms other than isolated posterior leaflet prolapse has been associated with more complex and time-consuming repair methods and has been characterized by higher rates of recurrent MVI [1–4]. The "French correction" proposed by Carpentier certainly provided major breakthroughs for reconstructing the mitral valve in the presence of variable patterns of MVI [6], but postoperative results were indisputably less favorable for specific MVI settings like anterior, bileaflet, or commissural lesions [1–4]. Under these circumstances, the traditional repair techniques proposed were more complex and often not easily reproducible. More expeditious and reliable techniques were advocated by the surgical community to overcome the above mentioned drawbacks in the treatment of MVI. The edge-to-edge (EE) technique was therefore designed to provide a simple, quick, and reproducible procedure meant to restore durable mitral leaflet coaptation in several MVI patterns, but, particularly, to counteract anterior, bileaflet, or commissural-based prolapse and MV regurgitation [7].

R. Lorusso, MD, PhD (✉)
Cardiac Surgery Unit, Spedali Civili Hospital,
Piazzale Spedali Civili, 1, Brescia 25123, Italy
e-mail: ro.lorusso@libero.it

E. Vizzardi, MD
Cardiology Unit, Spedali Civili Hospital,
Piazzale Spedali Civili, 1, Brescia 25123, Italy
e-mail: enrico.vizzardi@tin.it

S. Gelsomino, MD, PhD
Cardiovascular Research Centre Maastricht, MUMC,
P. Debyelaan 25, Maastricht 6229, The Netherlands
e-mail: sandro.gelsomino@libero.it

© Springer International Publishing Switzerland 2015
O. Alfieri et al. (eds.), *Edge-to-Edge Mitral Repair: From a Surgical to a Percutaneous Approach*, DOI 10.1007/978-3-319-19893-4_6

This technique was initially applied in all spectra of mitral valve disease, with early encouraging results [7]. Subsequently, peculiar types of valve dysfunction showed less favorable outcomes highlighting the importance of careful patient selection to provide more durable results [8, 9]. In addition the importance of several technical details in performing the EE technique became more clear.

This chapter deals with such a "technique and knowledge-related EE journey" which emerged during and following the initial phase of this procedure. Better understanding of anatomical and functional details, assessment of clinical outcomes, simulation with computational models, and refinement of surgical details were all instrumental aspects for subsequent improvement of the EE operation for MVI.

## 6.1  First Clinical Experiences and Subsequent Insights for Refined EE

The EE technique was introduced into clinical practice in 1991 with the first clinical experience reported in 1995, which included 35 patients reviewed during a 3-year follow-up time [7]. The subsequent more extensive experience was reported in 1998 consisting of 121 patients with a freedom from reoperation of 95 % ± 4.8 % at 6 years, and with 91 % of the patients with no or trivial mitral regurgitation (MR) and a mean valve area of $3.0 \pm 0.97$ cm$^2$ [8]. In this early adoption phase, the EE was used to treat variable MVI pathologies, from degenerative to rheumatic, including acute endocarditis and ischemic regurgitation. The EE procedure appeared to be an appealing technique which was able to provide a versatile, rapid, and effective repair in complex scenarios. The increasing experience led to clinical as well as laboratory investigations, including computational models, in order to address several aspects of the surgical technique. The information gathered have been able to address some specific concerns about the EE procedure and to define some drawbacks or peculiar management in specific disease environments, with paramount impact on long-term results.

### 6.1.1  Safety of EE Approximating Stitch

The first issue elucidated by the very first relevant clinical experiences [7–15] was that breakdown of the approximating suture occurred in very few patients, as shown by only one patient in the Cleveland Clinic report [10], one case due to early acute endocarditis in the Brescia experience [7, 12, 13, 15], and none (0 %) in the Milan series [8, 9, 11, 14]. This important information reassured the surgical community that such a procedure could be safely performed, with no tearing of the approximated leaflets and, hence, no early, premature, or sudden recurrence of MVI. Small pericardial or Teflon pledgets were initially applied to reduce mechanical tension on the sutured edges, particularly in presence of fibroelastic deficiency [7, 8, 12]. The existence of increased stresses close to the EE suture was confirmed by computational models [16–18]. In addition, computer simulation demonstrated that the adjunct of an annuloplasty ring was able to reduce significantly the tension on the approximated edges [17, 18]. These data were elegantly confirmed by Timek and associates [19] who showed in an animal model of the EE that, in the absence of a prosthetic ring, annular size was the primary determinant of the tension exerted on the approximated segments. This observation confirmed the need of an associated annuloplasty procedure to provide a more durable EE repair [9, 11]. On the other hand, increased contractility achieved with dobutamine infusion was able to decrease the leaflet tension, indicating that enhanced coaptation does reduce the stress exerted on the sutured leaflets [19].

## 6.1.2  EE Suture Width and Mitral Valve Stenosis

Leaflet approximation was achieved, from the beginning, with a running suture, and the width of such a forced coaptation was at the beginning meant just to enhance leaflet opposition, eliminating single or bileaflet prolapse. The EE suture has the precise objective to address the prolapsing segments of the dysfunctional leaflets. In the presence of a Barlow valve, however, it might be used also to reduce the redundant tissue participating to the MV mechanics. The concern about the residual valve area, however, was since the beginning addressed by measuring the double-orifice surfaces through Hegar dilator application through the generated orifices, thereby obtaining accurate valve measurement. The availability of a two-orifice area superior to 2.5 cm$^2$ was almost invariably achieved in all clinical series, guaranteeing the respect of a functionally and hemodynamically acceptable MV opening and unrestricted blood flow. In more than 800 patients, only two cases of EE repair failure due to valve stenosis were recorded [7–15] and both during the very initial experiences, suggesting that this concern does not represent an actual shortcoming of such a surgical technique.

## 6.1.3  Annuloplasty and EE

The use of associated annuloplasty became increasingly evident as another determinant of the EE results. The presence of a prosthetic ring, mainly complete, proved to provide essential stability and reduced mechanical tension on the approximated spot and nearby leaflet segments [9, 11, 13, 15–19]. Jimenez and colleagues clearly showed, in an ex vivo model of fresh porcine MVs instrumented in a pulsatile apparatus and with tension transducer applied at the approximating suture, that the presence of annular dilatation may negatively affect EE MV correction [20]. The use of an annuloplasty represents another step in the evolution of such MVR and is currently an important procedural detail.

## 6.1.4  Systolic Anterior Motion (SAM) and EE

The impact of the EE on the occurrence of SAM of the repaired MV also soon appeared favorable. Indeed, such an adverse event after MVR was rarely recorded in the EE clinical series. As a matter of fact, the EE proved to be an optimal solution in case of SAM development, as shown by Mascagni and colleagues [21]. In this series, the application of the EE in four patients, who experienced SAM after MVR due to posterior MV leaflet prolapse without chordal rupture, was capable of solving the hemodynamic and anatomical dysfunction with total disappearance of SAM immediately after MVR. Interestingly, this action was also maintained at long-term [21].

### 6.1.5   EE as a Bail-out Procedure for Intraoperatively Failed Conventional MVRs

After having confirmed that the EE technique was a reproducible, reliable, and easy-to perform operation to treat several patterns of MVI, it came out that it could represent an effective bail-out procedure in case of complex conventional MVRs failed intraoperatively [22]. Brinster and coworkers described an initial series of 52 patients in whom the EE technique was used as a bail-out procedure in presence of residual regurgitation and/or SAM after conventional reparative techniques [23]. Particularly in patients with post-repair SAM, the rescue EE was very effective both perioperatively and at long term. Similar findings were reported by De Bonis and coworkers who confirmed the very good durability at long-term of a similar approach to save mitral valves with a less than satisfactory result after a standard reconstructive method [22].

### 6.1.6   Mitral Valve Pathologies and EE

#### 6.1.6.1 Infective Endocarditis
The EE proved to be feasible and effective also in particularly difficult conditions, like acute endocarditis. Extensive free margin excision for infective involvement or vegetectomy may still allow the application of leaflet approximation to ensure valve preservation and adequate leaflet coaptation [24]. The use of EE in such a context, however, must be balanced with the need of radical excision of the infected tissue. On the other hand, its application in healed endocarditis has shown to portend favorable early and long-term outcome [7, 9, 10] and should be considered whenever the anatomical features allow it.

#### 6.1.6.2 Secondary MVI
In the initial experience the use of the EE in ischemic MVI appeared to be promising [7, 9]. The impact of MVR in post-infarction MVI is a well known ongoing debate, and all the MVR techniques have shown to provide limited benefit at mid and long term [25]. The limited effect of isolated EE technique without annulo-pasty in the presence of acute ischemic mitral regurgitation was elegantly shown by Timek and co-workers in an animal model. Indeed the EE stitch, without any intervention on the mitral annulus, did not influence the severity of acute MR and did not improve the geometrical alteration induced by the ischemic insult on the subvalvular apparatus [19]. The actual benefit of the EE repair in functional and, in

particular, in ischemic MVI, has been controversial and also questioned [10], but several clinical series have shown favorable mid and long-term results, particularly in patients with postoperative reverse remodelling [26, 27]. In many patients, the EE is capable to immediately abolish MVI by forcefully reversing leaflet tethering with the approximating stitch. However, despite the stabilizing effect of the annular ring and the central or paracommissural stitches, progressive ventricular dilatation or myocardial wall akinesia or dyskinesia may perpetuate tethering forces also on an EE reconstructed valve, possibly inducing recurrent MVI laterally to the EE stitch. Ongoing studies evaluating the feasibility and efficacy of the percutaneous EE in patients with depressed left ventricular function and ischemic MVI will likely provide further meaningful information for enhanced management of these patients.

### 6.1.6.3 Rheumatic MVI
As with other MV pathologies, the EE procedure showed clear limitations in rheumatic mitral disease [9, 13]. Thickened or partially calcified leaflet are definitely not suitable for such a technique.

### 6.1.6.4 Fibroelastic Deficiency
The EE was also debated in the setting of fibroelastic deficiency. In this situation, usually the MV presents thin leaflets and no tissue redundancy, making the EE technique less applicable or appealing, with concerns about the risk of approximating stitch breakdown. As mentioned, the EE was applied in several cases of fibroelastic deficiency and no case of premature or early rupture of the suture were recorded indicating that appropriate approximation and, maybe, the adjunct of supportive pledgets may be helpful in these circumstances.

### 6.1.6.5 Uncommon Scenarios
The use of the EE in other difficult, or peculiar cardiac or surgical conditions was pointed out by several investigators. Sartipy and associates have shown the use of such an MVR in patients undergoing left ventricular restoration [28]. This approach was also applied by the Cleveland Clinic group in 48 patients, 20 of whom had a transventricular EE [10]. It must be underlined that performing an EE procedure in these circumstances may limit the MVR success if an annuloplasty is not concomitantly applied as repeatedly demonstrated. An annular ring, either partial or complete, however, has been shown to be possible in some of those uncommon instances [29, 30]. A transaortic approach to perform the EE has been also shown and may represent a useful tool in case of difficult atrial access while performing aortic valve or ascending aorta procedures [31, 32].

## 6.1.7  EE in Barlow Valves with Excessive Redundant Tissue

It became soon clear that addressing the so called "Barlow valves" was not a major issue, rather, the possibility to achieve bileaflet approximation with generous suturing bites in these circumstances allowed the achievement of several objectives: the

**Fig. 6.1** Measurement of
mitral valve area with Hegar
dilators following an
edge-to-edge with triple-
orifice correction to address a
multiple-jet mitral valve
regurgitation is shown. Three
different orifices are obtained
as shown by three different
Hegar dimensions

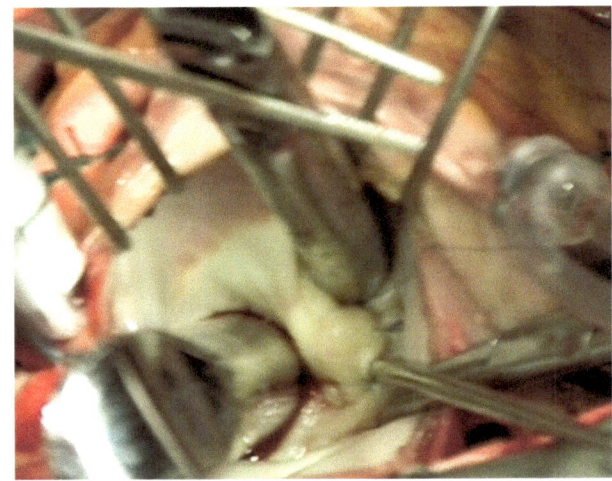

avoidance of leaflet resection, the use of leaflet tissue redundancy and strength for leaflet apposition, and the prevention of excessive valve area reduction. Indeed, the myxomatous valve features showed to be remarkably favorable for the EE procedure. Prompt MVI resolution could be achieved with a rather quick and simple surgical manoeuvre used in place of other more time-consuming and complex valve reconstruction. Moreover, the well known risk of SAM was also concomitantly addressed and avoided by the inherent configuration of the final EE valve, which effectively impedes or highly limits redundant leaflet motion toward the interventricular septum.

## 6.1.8   EE Repair in the Presence of Multiple-Jet MVI

The EE technique is usually extremely favorable in the treatment of MVI with a single regurgitant jet since the leaflet approximation is usually carried out just at the jet site, thereby addressing the culprit dysfunction of the valve anomaly. In case of multiple jets, the EE, by addressing the dominant lesion, in combination with the annular ring, is usually capable to remarkably reduce or abolish also the secondary jets. There are cases, however, in which more than one hemodynamically relevant jet are present, namely in extreme Barlow valves, with massive redundant tissue and significant annular dilatation. In these cases, an isolated EE plus annular ring might not be sufficient to counteract all the valve leaks. The adoption of a double EE suture has been therefore proposed [33] with the aim of addressing the two main regurgitant jets. This "triple-orifice" technique (Figs. 6.1, 6.2, and 6.3) is completed with the application of a complete annular ring which is usually effective in abolishing the single or multiple minor jets. The preliminary experience of 25 cases of these complex valve dysfunction with multiple hemodynamically

**Fig. 6.2** Triple-orifice edge-to-edge repair with ring implantation. The two approximating stitches reinforced with autologous pericardial patches are visible at the coaptation line

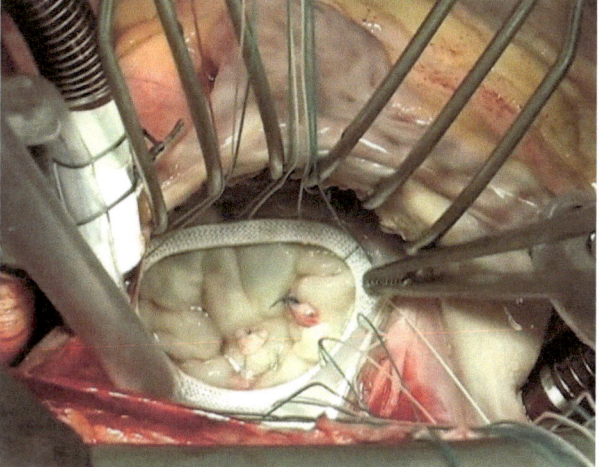

**Fig. 6.3** Intraoperative transesophageal ecocardiography showing the three transmitral flow jets after a triple-orifice edge-to-edge mitral valve repair

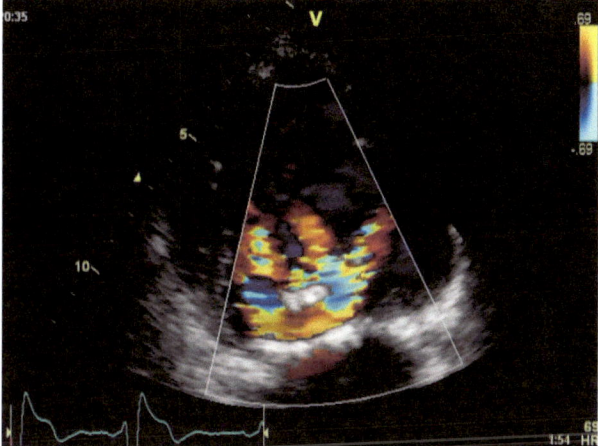

significant jets and treated with the "triple-orifice" procedure has shown favorable mid-term results and, therefore, might be considered in these particular and difficult MVI patient subsets.

---

### Conclusions

The EE proved to be highly effective in patients with severe MVI in several MV dysfunctional patterns and pathologies, with very few exception which are actually shared also with conventional MVR techniques. Simplicity, rapidity of execution, constant reproducibility, and surgical versatility (single, bileaflet, central or commissural, single or multi-jet patterns) represent the unquestionable virtues of such a procedure. Of course specific technical details need to be carefully respected during the operation. The progressive better understanding of the EE technique-related mechanisms led to its reliable application and to very satisfactory long-term results in several MVI subsets. In addition it paved the way to minimally invasive and percutaneous approaches [34]. As always, in surgery, this surgical concept and procedure highlighted the well known statement that most of the time "the simpler the better."

## References

1. Enriquez-Sarano M, Schaff HV, Orszulak TA, Tajik AJ, Bailey KR, Frye RL. Valve repair improves the outcome of surgery for mitral regurgitation. Circulation. 1995;91: 1022–8.
2. Gillinov AM, Cosgrove DM, Blackstone EH, Diaz R, Arnold JH, Lytle BW, Smedira NG, Sabik JF, McCarthy PM, Loop FD. Durability of mitral valve repair for degenerative disease. J Thorac Cardiovasc Surg. 1998;116:734–43.
3. Cohn LH, Couper GS, Aranki SF, Rizzo RJ, Kinchla NM, Collins JJ. Long-term results of mitral valve reconstruction for regurgitation of the myxomatous mitral valve. J Thorac Cardiovasc Surg. 1994;107:143–51.
4. Alvarez JM, Deal CW, Loveridge K, Brennan P, Eisenberg R, Ward M, Bhattacharya K, Atkinson SJ, Choong C. Repairing the degenerative mitral valve: ten to fifteen-year follow-up. J Thorac Cardiovasc Surg. 1996;112:238–47.
5. Perier P, Stumpf J, Gotz C, Lakew F, Schneider A, Clausnizer B, Hacker R. Valve repair for mitral regurgitation caused by isolated prolapse of the posterior leaflet. Ann Thorac Surg. 1997;64:445–50.
6. Carpentier A. Cardiac valve surgery. The French correction. J Thorac Cardiovasc Surg. 1983;86:323–7.
7. Fucci C, Sandrelli L, Pardini A, Torracca L, Ferrari M, Alfieri O. Improved results with mitral valve repair using new surgical techniques. Eur J Cardiothorac Surg. 1995;9:621–7.
8. Maisano F, Torracca L, Oppizzi M, Stefano PL, D'Addario G, La Canna G, Zogno M, Alfieri O. The edge-to-edge technique: a simplified method to correct mitral insufficiency. Eur J Cardiothorac Surg. 1998;13(3):240–6.
9. Alfieri O, Maisano F, De Bonis M, Stefano PL, Torracca L, Oppizzi M, La Canna G. The double-orifice technique in mitral valve repair: a simple solution for complex problems. J Thorac Cardiovasc Surg. 2001;122:674–81.
10. Bhudia SK, McCarthy PM, Smedira NG, Lam BK, Rajeswaran J, Blackstone EH. Edge-to-edge (Afieri) mitral repair: results in diverse clinical settings. Ann Thorac Surg. 2004; 77:1598–606.
11. Maisano F, Caldarola A, Blasio A, De Bonis M, La Canna G, Alfieri O. Mid-term results of the edge-to-edge mitral valve repair without annuloplasty. J Thorac Cardiovasc Surg. 2003;126: 1987–97.
12. Totaro P, Tulumello E, Fellini P, Rambaldini M, Rocco D, Coletti G, Zogno M, Lorusso R. Mitral valve repair for isolated prolapse of the anterior leaflet: an eleven-year follow-up. Eur J Cardiothorac Surg. 1999;15:119–26.
13. Lorusso R, Borghetti V, Totaro P, Parrinello G, Coletti G, Minzioni G. The double-orifice technique for mitral valve reconstruction: predictors of postoperative outcome. Eur J Cardiothorac Surg. 2001;20:583–9.
14. Maisano F, Schreuder JJ, Oppizzi M, Fiorani B, Fino C, Alfieri O. The double-orifice technique as a standardized approach to treat mitral regurgitation due to severe myxomatous disease. Eur J Cardiothorac Surg. 2000;17:201–5.
15. Borghetti V, Campana M, Scotti C, Domenighini D, Totaro P, Coletti G, Pagani M, Lorusso R. Biological versus prosthetic ring in mitral valve repair : enhancement of mitral annulus dynamics and left ventricular function with pericardial annuloplasty at long term. Eur J Cardiothorac Surg. 2000;17:431–9.

16. Maisano F, Redaelli A, Pennati G, Fumero R, Torracca L, Alfieri O. The hemodynamic effects of double-orifice valve repair for mitral regurgitation : a 3D computational model. Eur J Cardiothorac Surg. 1999;15:419–25.
17. Votta E, Maisano F, Soncini M, Redaelli A, Montevecchi FM, Alfieri O. 3-D computational analysis of the stress distribution on the leaflets after edge-to-edge repair of mitra regurgitation. J Heart Valve Dis. 2002;11:810–22.
18. Dal Pan F, Donzella G, Fucci C, Schreiber M. Structural effects of an innovative surgical technique to repair heart valve defects. J Biomech. 2005;38:2460–71.
19. Timek TA, Nielsen AL, Lai DT, Tibayan FA, Liang D, Rodriguez F, Daughters GT, Ingels NB, Miller CD. Edge-to-edge mitral valve repair without ring annuloplasty for acute ischemic mitral regurgitation. Circulation. 2003;108(Suppl II):II–122.
20. Jimenez JH, Forbess J, Croft LR, Small L, He Z, Yoganathan AP. Effects of annular size, transmitral pressure, and mitral flow rate on the Edge-To-Edge repair: an in-vitro study. Ann Thorac Surg. 2006;82:1362–8.
21. Mascagni R, Al Attar N, Lamarra M, Calvi S, Tripodi A, Mebazaa A, Lessana A. Edge-to-edge technique to treat post-mitral valve repair systolic anterior motion and left ventricular outflow tract obstruction. Ann Thorac Surg. 2005;79:471–4.
22. De Bonis M, Lapenna E, Buzzatti N, Taramasso M, Calabrese MC, Nisi T, Pappalardo F, Alfieri O. Can the edge-to-edge technique provide durable results when used to rescue patients with suboptimal conventional mitral repair? Eur J Cardiothorac Surg. 2013;43(6):e173–9.
23. Brinster DR, Unic D, D'Ambra MN, Nathan N, Cohn LH. Midterm results of the Edge-to-Edge technique for complex mitral valve repair. Ann Thorac Surg. 2006;81:1612–7.
24. Lorusso R, Fucci C, Pentiricci S, Coletti G, La Canna G, Zogno M. "Double-orifice" technique to repair extensive mitral valve excision following acute endocarditis. J Card Surg. 1998;13:24–6.
25. Lorusso R, Gelsomino S, Vizzardi E, D'Aloia A, De Cicco G, Lucà F, Parise O, Gensini GF, Stefàno PL, Livi U, Vendramin I, Pacini D, Di Bartolomeo R, Miceli A, Glauber M, Varone E, Parolari A, Alamanni F, Serraino F, Renzulli A, Messina A, Troise G, Mariscalco G, Beghi C, Nicolini F, Gherli T, Borghetti V, Pardini A, Caimmi PP, Micalizzi E, Fino C, Ferrazzi P, Di Mauro M. Calafiore. Mitral valve repair or replacement for ischemic mitral regurgitation ? The Italian Study on Treatment of Ischemic mitral Regurgitation (ISTMIR). J Thorac Cardiovasc Surg. 2013;145:128–39.
26. De Bonis M, Ferrara D, Taramasso M, Calabrese MC, Verzini A, Buzzatti N, Alfieri O. Mitral valve replacement or repair for functional mitral valve regurgitation in dilated and ischemic cardiomyopathy: is it really the same? Ann Thorac Surg. 2012;94:44–51.
27. Kuduvalli M, Ghotkar SV, Grayson AD, Fabri BM. Edge-to-edge technique for mitral valve repair: medium-term results with echocardiographic follow-up. Ann Thorac Surg. 2006;82:1356–61.
28. Sartipy U, Albage A, Mattsson E, Lindblom D. Edge-to-edge mitral repair without annuloplasty in combination with surgical ventricular restoration. Ann Thorac Surg. 2007;83:1303–9.
29. Mc Carthy PM, Starling RC, Wong J, Scalia GM, Buda T, Vargo RL, Goormastic M, Thomas JD, Smedira NG, Young JB. Early results with partial left ventriculectomy. J Thorac Cardiovasc Surg. 1997;114:755–65.
30. Batista RJ, Verde J, Nery P, Bocchino L, Takeshita N, Bhayana JN, Bergsland J, Graham S, Houck JP, Salerno TA. Partial left ventriculectomy to treat end-stage heart disease. Ann Thorac Surg. 1997;64:634–8.
31. Kallner G, van der Linden J, Hadjinikolau L, Lindblom D. Transaortic approach for the Alfieri stitch. Ann Thorac Surg. 2001;71:378–9.
32. Kavarana MN, Edwards NM, Levinson MM, Oz MC. Transaortic repair of mitral regurgitation. Heart Surg Forum. 2000;3:24–8.
33. Fucci C, Faggiano P, Nardi M, D'Aloia A, Coletti G, De Cicco G, Latini L, Vizzardi E, Lorusso R. Triple-orifice repair in severe Barlow disease with multiple-jet mitral regurgitation: report of mid-term results. Int J Cardiol. 2013;167:2623–9.
34. De Bonis M, Lapenna E, Maisano F, Barili F, La Canna G, Buzzatti N, Pappalardo F, Calabrese M, Nisi T, Alfieri O. Long-term results (≤18 years) of the edge-to-edge mitral valve repair without annuloplasty in degenerative mitral regurgitation: implications for the percutaneous approach. Circulation. 2014;130(Suppl I):S19–24.

# Results of the Edge-to-Edge Mitral Valve Repair

7

Michele De Bonis, Elisabetta Lapenna,
Gabriele Del Castillo, and Ottavio Alfieri

## 7.1    Introduction

After its introduction in the early 90s, the edge-to-edge (EE) technique has been used in patients with mitral regurgitation (MR) due to different etiologies and mechanisms [1–7]. However, clinical and echocardiographic results have progressively demonstrated suboptimal results in patients with rheumatic valve disease and in those who did not receive a concomitant annuloplasty procedure [2, 8]. In the above mentioned conditions, the EE repair does not represent the technique of choice and, after the early experience, it has been progressively abandoned. More than 20 years after its introduction, it is now clear that the best indications for the EE repair are represented by bileaflet prolapse (facing segments), segmental anterior leaflet prolapse/flail and commissural prolapse/flail. In addition this technique does have an important role also in functional mitral regurgitation, and as a "rescue" procedure in case of suboptimal conventional mitral reconstruction ("rescue" EE). Finally it has been used for the prevention/treatment of SAM (in HOCM or following mitral repair) and, occasionally, in some cases of complex congenital atrio-ventricular valve incompetence. In this chapter the results of the EE repair in the most common indications described above will be outlined and discussed.

## 7.2    Bileaflet Prolapse of Facing Segments in Barlow's Disease

In patients with a global mixomatous degeneration of the mitral valve (Barlow's disease), all the components of the mitral apparatus are affected by a pathologic process which leads to generalized bileaflet prolapse and severe annular

M. De Bonis, MD (✉) • E. Lapenna • G. Del Castillo • O. Alfieri
Department of Cardiac Surgery, IRCCS San Raffaele University Hospital, Milan, Italy
e-mail: debonis.michele@hsr.it

© Springer International Publishing Switzerland 2015
O. Alfieri et al. (eds.), *Edge-to-Edge Mitral Repair: From a Surgical to a Percutaneous Approach*, DOI 10.1007/978-3-319-19893-4_7

dilatation. In most of the cases, however, the prolapse involves mainly the facing segments of the central portions of the anterior and posterior leaflets (A2 and P2) making it possible the surgical correction of MR by the EE technique. By suturing the middle scallop of the anterior and posterior leaflet (A2 to P2) followed by ring annuloplasty, the EE restores valve competence [9], reduces the height of the leaflets in their middle portion and lowers the level of coaptation below the annulus.

Mid-term results in the first 82 patients demonstrated that the EE technique could be effectively adopted with a very short aortic cross-clamp time ($38 \pm 12$ min) [9]. In only one patient, the total valve area, measured with Hegar dilators immediately after the procedure, was less than 2.0 cm$^2$ and valve replacement had to be performed. None of the remaining patients had postoperative mitral stenosis. The mean postoperative valve area, assessed by trans-esophageal Doppler echocardiography, was $3.7 \pm 0.79$ cm$^2$ (against a mean preoperative value of $9.2 \pm 2.1$ cm$^2$). At hospital discharge, no or mild regurgitation was found in all but three patients who showed moderate residual regurgitation. Freedom from reoperation was $86 \pm 14$ % at 5 years.

Those data confirmed the efficacy of the double-orifice repair as a standardized approach to treat valve regurgitation due to Barlow's disease. However, they were limited by the rather short follow-up time, which allowed drawing conclusions just at mid-term. More recently, the long-term clinical and echocardiographic outcomes of this approach have been described in the first 128 patients (mean EF $60 \pm 4.5$ %) who had been treated with a double orifice EE repair between the years 1993 and 2000 in our centre [10]. All patients underwent a concomitant prosthetic ring annuloplasty (mean size of the ring $36.6 \pm 2.5$ mm). Mean clinical follow-up was $11.5 \pm 2.53$ years (range 1.1–17.6 years) and more than 95 % of the patients underwent an echocardiographic exam at this time. Freedom from reoperation at 14 years was $90.6. \pm 2.96$ %. Mitral stenosis requiring reoperation was detected in only one patient (1/128 patients, 0.7 %). All the other reoperations were performed because of severe recurrent MR. At 12 years freedom from recurrence of MR $\geq$ 3+ was $86.3 \pm 3.54$ % (Fig. 7.1). The only predictor of recurrence of MR $\geq$ 3+ at follow-up was residual regurgitation greater than mild at hospital discharge ($p = 0.007$) confirming the importance of a perfectly competent mitral valve at the end of the reconstructive procedure. In a number of patients the mechanism responsible for recurrent MR remained unclear, either because reoperations were performed in other Institutions or because this information was not described in detail in the operative reports. However, in those patients in whom the cause of recurrence of MR could be established, this was usually due to progression of the degenerative disease with the occurrence of new prolapsing or flailing lesions in correspondence of one of the two orifices of the EE repair. Tearing of the leaflet by the EE suture occurred only in one case together with prosthetic ring detachment. An interesting finding was that none of the patient required reoperation for postoperative SAM demonstrating that, if the EE suture is performed with deep bites in order to decrease

**Fig. 7.1** Long-term freedom from recurrence of MR ≥ 3+ in patients treated with double orifice EE repair for bileaflet prolapse (BLP: bileaflet prolapse)

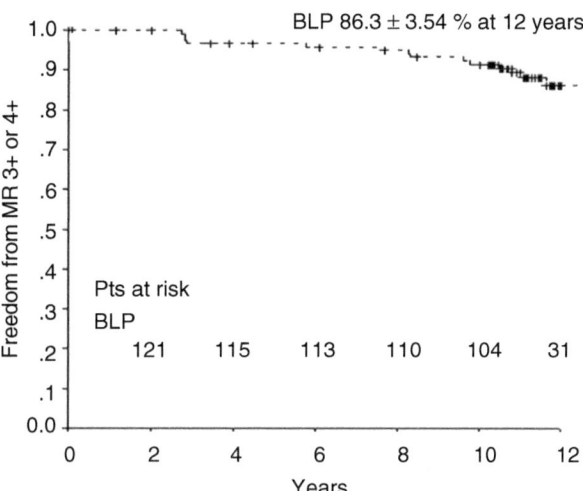

the height of the leaflets, a postoperative SAM can be effectively prevented. Finally a significant clinical improvement was documented at follow-up with more than 95 % of the patients in NYHA functional class I or II. All together those clinical and echocardiographic results are at least comparable if not better than those described in other series with similar follow-up length [11–14] and confirm that the double orifice technique, combined with ring annuloplasty, provides excellent late outcomes in patients with degenerative MR and bileaflet prolapse. Besides the freedom from reoperation, the echocardiographic controls at follow-up have definitively proved the long-term effectiveness and durability of this method of repair in this challenging setting.

## 7.3  Segmental Prolapse of the Anterior Leaflet

A very good indication for the EE technique is represented by severe MR due to segmental prolapse of the anterior leaflet in the setting of degenerative MV pathology (mixomatous disease or fibroelastic deficiency) or post-endocarditis MR. If only one scallop is prolapsing, the EE repair is very effective in restoring MV competence in a rapid, standardized and easily reproducible manner. Also in this setting the long-term clinical and echocardiographic results are now available for the first 139 patients treated with this approach in our centre [15]. All patients had severe degenerative MR due to isolated segmental prolapse/flail of the anterior leaflet and underwent EE repair combined with annuloplasty. Mean age was 54 ± 14.4 years and 68.9 % of the patients were in NYHA class I–II. Mean LVEF was 56 ± 7.8 % and 28 (20.1 %) were in atrial fibrillation. In 105 patients (75.5 %) with prolapse or flail of A2, the EE suture was placed in (or close to) the central portion of the leaflets

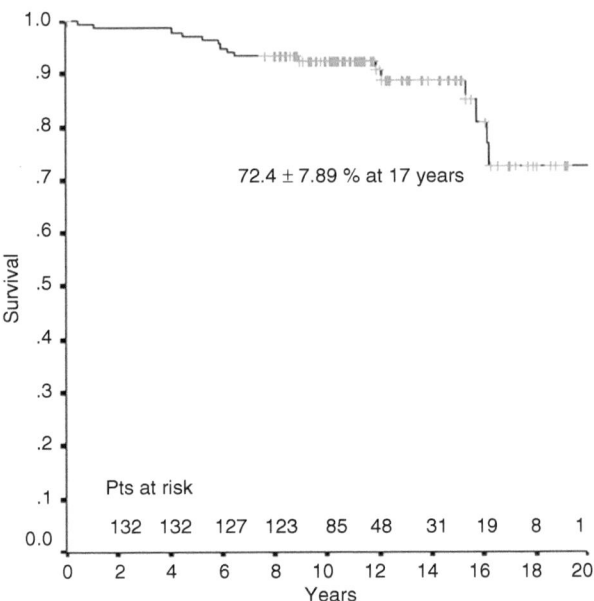

**Fig. 7.2** Overall survival in patients treated with the EE repair for anterior leaflet prolapse (Reprinted with permission from [15])

(double orifice repair), while in 34 patients (24.5 %) with either A1 or A3 lesions, the approximation of the free edges of the leaflets was carried out in continuity with the commissure (paracommissural repair). The concomitant annuloplasty procedure was performed with a prosthetic ring in the vast majority of cases (92 %) while a posterior annuloplasty with autologous pericardium was preferred in 11 (8 %) patients. Only four patients were lost to follow-up which was therefore 97.1 % complete. The mean length of follow-up was 11.5±3.73 years (up to 21.5 years). There were no hospital deaths. At 17 years the actuarial overall survival was 72±7.89 (Fig. 7.2) and freedom from cardiac death was 90±4.73 % (Fig. 7.3). Thirteen patients were reoperated for severe MR between 1 month and 9 years after the initial repair. Freedom from reoperation at 17 years was 89.6±2.74 % (Fig. 7.4).

At the last echocardiogram, mean mitral valve area was 2.9±0.46 cm² (median 3 cm², range 1.8–4 cm²). Clinically relevant mitral stenosis was never detected. Overall 17 patients (12.5 %) had recurrent MR ≥3+ at follow-up. Freedom from MR 3+ or 4+ at 17 years was 80.2±5.86 % (Fig. 7.5). At multivariate analysis, the only independent predictor of recurrence of MR ≥ 3+ was residual MR greater than mild at hospital discharge (HR 7.4, 95 % CI 2.5–21.2, $P=0.0001$) although the use of posterior pericardial rather than prosthetic ring annuloplasty was very close to the statistical significance as well (HR 2.8, 95 % CI 0.9–8.7, $P=0.06$).

A significant clinical improvement was also documented. Indeed NYHA class I was present in 94 patients (69.6 %), NYHA class II in 35 (25.9 %) and NYHA class III in 6 (4.4 %) ($P=0.0001$ compared to preoperative values).

**Fig. 7.3** Freedom from cardiac death in patients treated with the EE repair for anterior leaflet prolapse (Reprinted with permission from [15])

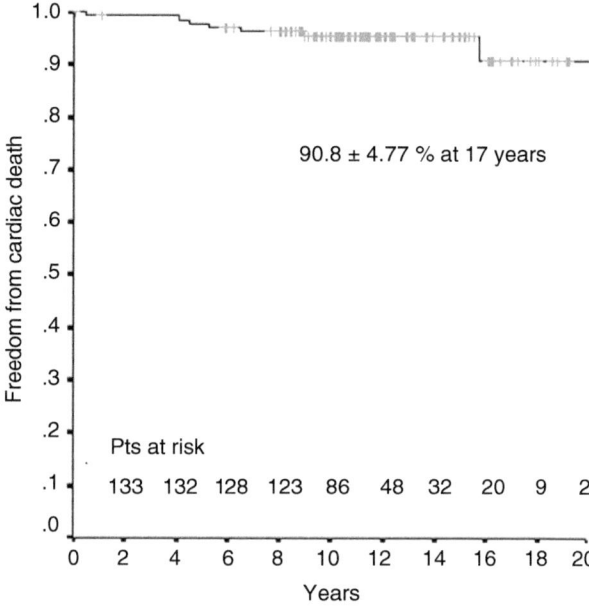

**Fig. 7.4** Freedom from reoperation in patients treated with the EE repair for anterior leaflet prolapse (Reprinted with permission from [15])

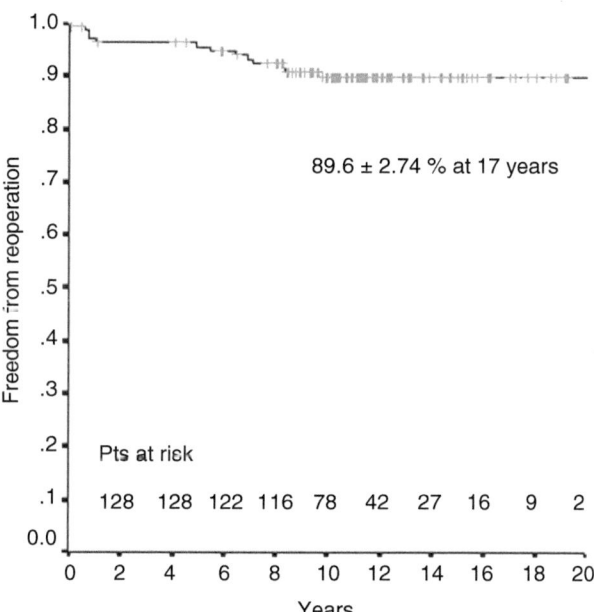

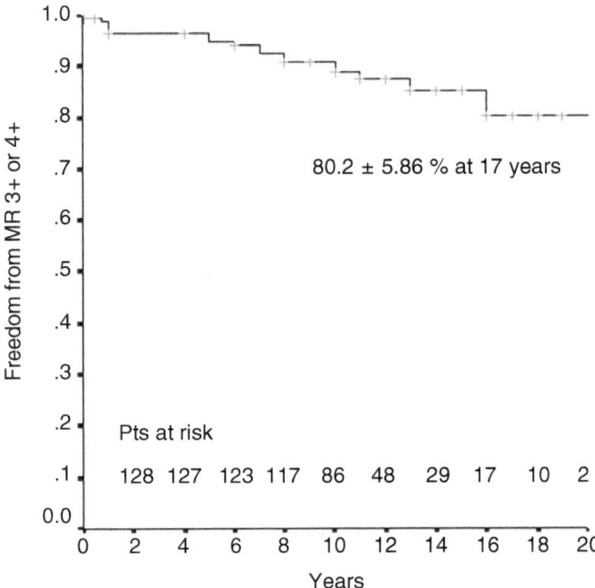

**Fig. 7.5** Freedom from recurrence of MR 3+ or 4+ in patients treated with the EE repair for anterior leaflet prolapse (Reprinted with permission from [15])

Those long-term clinical and echocardiographic data confirm that the EE mitral valve repair, combined with annuloplasty, provides excellent long-term results in patients with degenerative MR in the setting of segmental anterior leaflet prolapse. They also show that an immediate perfect result is essential to achieve optimal late durability. Those findings at late follow-up are very important because, unlike posterior leaflet prolapse, the prolapse of the anterior leaflet has been traditionally associated with decreased repair rate [16–18] and higher MR recurrence, even in experienced centres and with several different surgical techniques [19–21]. The EE approach preferentially adopted in our Institution provided excellent results at mid-term [22], which was then confirmed both clinically and echocardiographically at a median interval of 11 years after surgery [15]. The 90 % freedom from reoperation at 17 years observed in our experience is excellent and compares favourably with that reported by other groups using conventional repair techniques and with a duration of follow-up ranging from 10 to 20 years [11, 14, 20, 23]. Moreover, a strength of this study is that the predictability of the EE technique was demonstrated not only by the low incidence of reoperations, but also by the echocardiographic examinations. Nevertheless we recognize that, in presence of extended prolapse of the anterior leaflet, involving more than one scallop, the EE technique alone may not be sufficient to obtain a perfectly competent valve since a long suture would be required and mitral stenosis would likely be created. In those circumstances, other techniques should be preferred or artificial chordae should be added to the EE repair in order to eliminate incompetence without excessively reducing the mitral valve area.

## 7.4   Commissural Prolapse

In patients with severe MR due to commissural chordal rupture or elongation, several methods of repair have been suggested including neochordae implantation, chordal transposition, extended leaflet sliding technique, papillary muscle repositioning [24–26]. The absence of a unique and standardized approach in this context demonstrates the challenging feature of "commissural MR" which can be due to the pathologic involvement of the anterior, posterior or both leaflets. A technical solution tailored to the specific mechanism is usually required but the conventional surgical procedures can be challenging for a number of reasons: judgement of artificial chordal length can be difficult due to the fan-shaped anatomy of the commissural chordae; chordal reimplantation/transposition is not easy because of the fragility of commissural chordae; leaflet resection combined with an extended sliding carries the risk of distortion of the subvalvular apparatus; papillary muscle repositioning requires manipulation of the subvalvular apparatus and many surgeons have little confidence with it. Unlike those methods, the EE approximation of the anterior and posterior leaflet along the entire commissural area of prolapse (paracommissural EE) effectively eliminates MR simply and rapidly, regardless of the fact that the anterior, posterior or both leaflets are involved. Suturing both leaflets together raises a number of questions regarding the risk of inducing mitral stenosis, the degree of impairment of mitral leaflet motion and the overall long-term durability. However, the data accumulated so far show that the supposed drawbacks and risks of this technique are more theoretical than practical since no significant restriction has been demonstrated and durable results have been documented [27–29]. In the Cleveland Clinic experience, more than 100 patients with commissural prolapse/ flail were treated with suture closure of the commissure, with no instances of mitral stenosis, suture dehiscence or recurrent prolapse in the follow-up [27]. Similar results were found in our Institution [28, 29]. In a series of 125 patients followed at long-term [29], the etiology of commissural MR was degenerative in 89 % of the cases and post-endocarditis in the remaining 11 %. According to the location of the regurgitant jet, the EE was performed in correspondence of the postero-medial (77 %) or antero-lateral commissure (23 %). An annuloplasty was added to complete the repair. There were two hospital deaths (1.6 %). At hospital discharge a TTE was performed in all hospital survivors: MR was absent or mild in 120 (97.5 %) patients and moderate (2+/4+) in 3 (2.4 %).

At long-term, from a clinical point of view, 11-year freedom from cardiac death was excellent (95.2 ± 3.3 %). About one forth of the patients were in NYHA class III or IV before surgery whereas at follow-up all patients were in functional class I or II confirming the positive clinical impact of the repair procedure. The overall incidence of re-operations and recurrence of significant MR (3+ or 4+) were extremely low. Freedom from reoperation was at 11 years 97.4 ± 1.4 % (Fig. 7.6) and from recurrent MR ≥3+ 96.3 ± 1.7 % (Fig. 7.7). Preoperative factors like age, sex, LV function, cardiac rhythm and severity of symptoms were not identified as predictors of recurrence of MR. Similarly the etiology of MR, the involvement of the anterior, posterior or both leaflets in the mechanism of MR and the location of

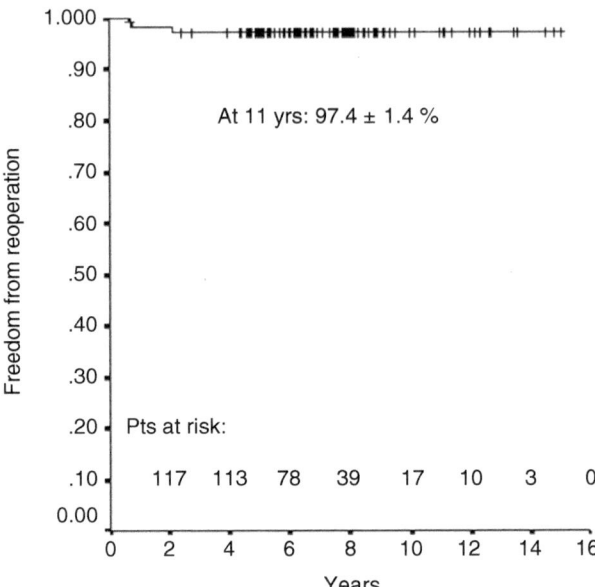

**Fig. 7.6** Freedom from reoperation in patients treated with the EE repair for commissural MR (Reprinted with permission from [29])

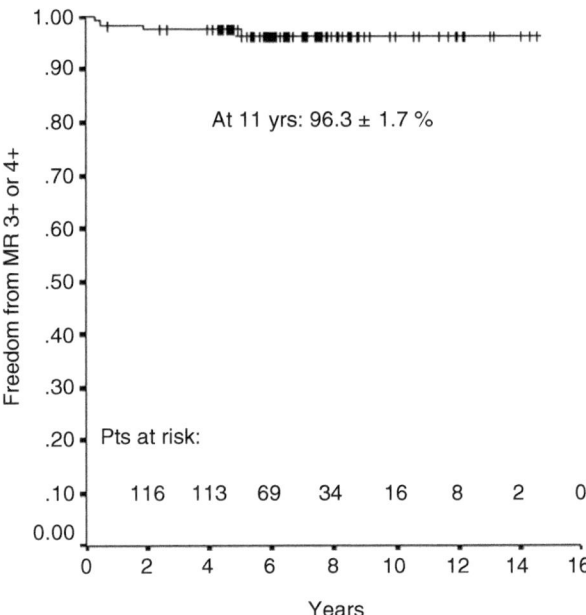

**Fig. 7.7** Freedom from recurrence of MR 3+ or 4+ in patients treated with the EE repair for commissural MR (Reprinted with permission from [29])

the regurgitant jet had no influence on the failure of the repair. Those long-term results are certainly very satisfactory considering that commissural prolapse is commonly believed to be a difficult lesion to treat. This "functional" rather than "anatomical" repair does not cause any significant restriction. This is confirmed by the low transvalvular pressure gradients recorded immediately after surgery as well as at the last echocardiographic follow-up. Indeed, at the last echocardiogram, mean mitral valve area and gradient were respectively $2.9 \pm 0.4$ cm$^2$ and $3.4 \pm 1.1$ mmHg (median 3 mmHg).

## 7.5 Functional Mitral Regurgitation

The EE technique can play a role in the treatment of MR secondary to ischemic or idiopathic dilated cardiomyopathy. Undersized annuloplasty using a complete rigid ring is the standard operation in functional MR. However several echocardiographic variables have been identified as predictors of failure of an isolated restrictive annuloplasty [30]. In presence of one or more predictors of failure of a restrictive annuloplasty, mitral valve replacement should be considered or, alternatively, other concomitant surgical procedures should be conveniently added according to the specific situation in order to enhance repair durability. The EE has been added to annuloplasty to enhance the likelihood of a durable repair in patients with more advanced degree of leaflets' tethering [31, 32]. The rationale for using the EE technique in functional MR is that, with this approach, the site of the regurgitant jet is specifically addressed, early valve closure is ensured and the occurrence of the "loitering effect" is abolished. Moreover, by anchoring the leaflets together, the EE might exert a kind of "reins" effect on the left ventricular chamber, counteracting the progression of the LV remodeling which can lead to recurrence of mitral regurgitation.

In our Institution the addition of the EE to annuloplasty in patients with a coaptation depth superior to 1 cm has been beneficial in decreasing the rate of residual or recurrent mitral regurgitation.

Since in functional MR the mitral valve is structurally normal, the intraoperative inspection does not provide additional information. The preoperative echocardiographic study, therefore, has literally to be used as a guide to identify the site of the approximating stitch which is chosen according to the echocardiographic location of the regurgitant jet. In case of central jet (between A2 and P2), a central EE repair is performed. On the other hand, when the regurgitant jet is in correspondence of the posterior commissure, as in some cases of ischemic MR, a commissural EE suture is applied. The length of the suture is always kept as short as possible to minimize the risk of postoperative mitral valve stenosis. A complete rigid or semirigid prosthetic ring is invariably implanted and, in secondary MR, it is usually one or two sizes smaller than the anterior leaflet surface. Our method of combining the "EE" technique with an undersized annuloplasty performed with a complete ring (preferentially rigid or semirigid), has resulted in a 3.7 % recurrence rate of 3 to 4+ MR at mid-term follow-up, which is sixfold lower compared to that registered in our centre with a restrictive annuloplasty alone (21.7 %) despite having, the EE patients, the more advanced degree of leaflet tethering [7]. Freedom from recurrence of severe MR at 1.5 years was 20 % higher in the EE group ($95 \pm 3.3$ % vs. $77 \pm 12.1$ %, respectively) [7]. Besides those mid-term outcomes, results at long-term have recently been obtained which confirmed a 9-year freedom from recurrence of MR $\geq$ 3+ of 86±5.6 % vs. 63±9.3 %, respectively ($P = 0.02$) (unpublished data). Failure or repair was associated with recurrence of NYHA 3 or 4 symptoms ($P < 0.0001$).

Further analysis of our overall experience with mitral repair in functional MR [33] identified the duration of CHF history as the only independent predictors of reverse LV remodelling at follow-up. It is worthy of mention the fact that the use of the EE technique showed a trend towards favouring reverse LV remodelling compared to isolated annuloplasty ($p = 0.08$) [33]. This finding could be explained by the fact that the EE technique, by anchoring the leaflets together, could exert a kind of "reins" effect on the LV chamber, counteracting the progression of the LV remodelling. This is extremely important considering that the occurrence of reverse remodelling is associated to longer repair durability and better clinical outcome [33, 34]. To exclude a restrictive effect, we measured the gradients at rest across the mitral valve after repair since the beginning of our experience. Both, immediately after surgery and at follow-up, they have been very low and a clinically relevant mitral stenosis has never been observed in any of the patients. Certainly, experience and careful choice of the annuloplasty ring and of the length of the EE suture are mandatory in order to avoid this risk. In addition, the EE technique should be avoided in the rare instances where severe leaflet tethering is associated with only mild annular dilatation since, in those cases, this method of repair would lead to a significant restrictive effect due to the lack of preoperative dilatation of the mitral annulus.

Other centres have been using the EE technique in patients with MR secondary to ischemic and idiopathic dilated cardiomyopathy. Encouraging [31], satisfactory [32] or disappointing results [5] have been described by those groups with this approach. Most of the unfavourable outcomes, however, have been reported when the EE technique has been employed without any concomitant annuloplasty [31] or in association with only a posterior flexible band [5, 31], which is unable to prevent the progression of annular dilatation in patients with dilated cardiomyopathy. In particular, the Cleveland Clinic group reported a disappointing 24 % recurrence rate of moderate-severe (3+/4+) mitral regurgitation 2 years after EE repair for functional mitral regurgitation [5]. However, in that series, the EE technique was always employed in association with a posterior flexible band and the patients requiring reoperation almost invariably presented re-dilatation of the mitral annulus. Moreover the EE suture was placed centrally in the great majority of the patients, regardless of the location of the regurgitant jet. Finally, there was no restriction in the use of the technique which was adopted also in presence of extreme degrees of left ventricular remodelling and tethering. In summary, the addition of the EE suture to a restrictive annuloplasty in patients with significant leaflets tethering (coaptation depth superior to 1 cm) has been beneficial in our experience, significantly improving the durability of the repair and showing a trend towards favouring reverse remodelling of the left ventricle. Of course unsatisfactory results can be expected even with the EE technique when the tethering of the leaflets is extreme and the degree of remodelling of the left ventricle is very important due to a long-lasting heart failure history. Under those circumstances mitral valve replacement or, in high surgical risk patients, a MitraClip implantation should be considered as the only suitable options to eliminate or, at least, improve functional MR.

## 7.6 The EE Technique to Prevent or Treat SAM

Systolic anterior motion (SAM) of the anterior mitral leaflet remains one of the most common complications after mitral valve repair. Although multiple surgical techniques have been proposed to prevent it, the overall prevalence of this event remains between 7 and 11 % [35]. It has been demonstrated that the use of the EE technique is effective in eliminating postoperative SAM in patients undergoing MV repair [4, 36]. Moreover recent data confirm that this method definitely has a role in preventing the occurrence of systolic anterior motion of the anterior MV leaflet in patients with pre-repair echocardiographic predictors of SAM [37].

Patients with hypertrophic obstructive cardiomyopathy (HOCM) and residual SAM after myectomy can also be cured by suturing together the anterior and posterior mitral leaflets, thereby completely eliminating any sign of left ventricular outflow tract (LVOT) obstruction [4, 38].

## 7.7 Rescue EE

An extremely interesting indication of the EE approach is represented by the use of this technique to "rescue" patients with significant residual MR after conventional mitral repair ("rescue EE" or "bailout EE"). The immediate result of any mitral valve reconstruction depends on a large number of variables including the etiology of MR, the complexity of the lesions, the quality of the preoperative echocardiographic diagnosis, the technique of repair and the surgical expertise. The goal of the repair is to achieve no or mild residual MR at the intraoperative trans-esophageal echocardiography and no SAM. However, 7–10 % of the patients do have a suboptimal immediate result after MV repair failure because of SAM, residual prolapse, inadequate annuloplasty, clefts and suture dehiscence [35–39]. In many instances the mechanism responsible for persistent regurgitation is clearly identified and can be easily corrected (residual clefts, suture dehiscence). In some patients, however, the cause of residual MR remains undefined or it would require time consuming conventional re-repair attempts (neochordae, further leaflet resection) to be addressed with an uncertain final result. Under those circumstances an additional EE suture can be added in correspondence of the site of the residual regurgitant jet without taking down the previous repair. Satisfactory results have been reported with this approach in a preliminary small group of patients [40]. We have adopted this solution in 43 patients with suboptimal conventional MV repair [41]. All 43 patients had either an unsatisfactory water test or a suboptimal result at the TEE control (SAM/residual MR $\geq$ 1+). In particular, a residual prolapse was observed in 30 patients (30/43, 69.7 %), refractory systolic anterior

motion in 12 (12/43, 27.9 %) and malcoaptation due to post-endocarditis leaflet ero-
sion in 1 (1/43, 2.3 %). Residual prolapse was usually the result of both misdiagnosis/
misinterpretation of the mechanisms of MR and wrong surgical decision making. A
rescue EE suture was performed in all cases without taking down the primary repair.
This technical solution was adopted whenever, in the opinion of the surgeon, a more
conventional re-repair would have been unsuitable or too time consuming or at high
risk of an unsatisfactory result.

The rescue EE was able to immediately restore valve competence in all
patients. The long-term durability of this approach was very satisfactory. During
the follow-up period, only one patient developed severe MR (treated with mitral
replacement) and 4 patients had moderate (2+/4+) mitral regurgitation, confirming a substantial stability of the repair. Freedom from $MR \geq 3+$ at 10 years was
$96.9 \pm 2.9$ %. One of the main advantages of the rescue EE is that it can be carried out with a short additional cross-clamp time ($15.2 \pm 5.6$ min in our series).
This is particularly important in patients who already had a long operation during the initial repair and in those with poor preoperative conditions or advanced
LV dysfunction. In addition, the "functional" rather than "anatomical" approach
provided by the EE technique allows the elimination of the residual regurgitant
jet regardless of the mechanism responsible for it. A potential drawback, on the
other hand, is the risk of inducing mitral stenosis considering that the original
MV area has already been reduced by the initial repair. That is the reason why,
in this setting, the suture has to be as short as possible (few millimeters) and
should probably be avoided in valves which have already a border-line residual
area after the first reconstruction. Significant mitral stenosis was never detected
in our patients either during the hospital stay or during follow-up as shown by
the low transvalvular gradients recorded. Most of the patients had a residual MV
area $\geq 2.5$ cm$^2$. Lower values (between 2 and 2.4 cm$^2$) were considered acceptable in eight patients with a small BSA ($\leq 1.6$ m$^2$). An exercise echocardiography to exclude functional mitral stenosis in those specific patients was not
performed. However, at a median follow-up of 5.4 years, the low mean transmitral gradient registered, the absence of pulmonary hypertension and the lack of
symptoms during exercise (NYHA class I) make the possibility of functional
mitral stenosis rather unlikely. In addition, Agricola and co-workers have previously demonstrated that patients with a MV area between 2 and 2.5 cm$^2$ after
double orifice EE repair combined with ring annuloplasty do not have any
important degree of mitral valve obstruction either at baseline or during physical exercise. Interestingly, the double orifice mitral valves with a smaller area at
rest demonstrate a higher capacity to increase their baseline area during exercise
compared to mitral valves with larger residual area [42]. In conclusion, the EE
technique can be an effective and durable option to restore valve competence
after a failed conventional repair. Mitral valves initially repaired with a

suboptimal result and then rescued with the adjunct of an EE suture remain competent at long-term.

## 7.8    The Role of Annuloplasty and the Risk of Stenosis

Absence of annuloplasty is associated with increased stresses on the suture and on the valve structure, leading to accelerated failure of the repair. As a matter of fact, in our clinical experience with the EE technique, freedom from reoperation was lower when annuloplasty was for some reasons omitted [2, 8]. A concomitant annuloplasty, therefore, represents a key factor for the long-term durability of the EE repair. In addition to the beneficial effects on the stresses exerted on the connecting suture and on the entire valve structures, the reduction of the annular size increases the coaptation surface of the leaflets and prevents subsequent annular dilatation.

Another relevant issue to be emphasized is the potential restrictive effect at rest and during exercise of a valve submitted to the EE repair. To address this issue, Frapier and co-workers [43] compared patients operated on either by Carpentier's techniques or by the EE repair. Rest and exercise echocardiogram along with cardiorespiratory testing with maximal oxygen uptake were performed. At baseline, the mean mitral valve area was 2.5 cm$^2$ after the EE and 2.9 cm$^2$ following classic mitral repair techniques ($p=0.0018$). However, despite the higher mitral valve area reduction, the EE technique did not induce more transvalvular gradients than classical Carpentier's repair (3.8 mmHg vs. 3.3 mmHg, respectively) ($P=$NS). At peak exercise, increase of the mitral gradient and maximum oxygen uptake (VO$_2$ max) was comparable between the two groups. This shows that the EE repair is no more restrictive at peak exercise than classic repairs and provides same exercise tolerance than Carpentier's techniques. In our Institution an exercise echocardiographic study was specifically designed to assess if the EE mitral repair could be a limiting factor for exercise tolerance. Thirty patients previously submitted to double orifice mitral valve repair, underwent exercise echocardiography (10 W per minute). At peak of the stress heart rate, systolic blood pressure and stroke volume significantly increased showing a physiologic behaviour of the mitral valve. The mean mitral valve gradient ($2.8\pm1.3$ mmHg vs. $4.6\pm1.9$ mmHg, $p<0.00001$), maximum mitral valve gradient ($6.4\pm2.8$ mmHg vs $10.5\pm4.6$ mmHg, $p<0.00002$) and systolic pulmonary artery pressure ($22.8\pm6.1$ mmHg vs $28.2\pm9.9$ mmHg, $p<0.001$) increased but not at pathologic levels. Planimetric valve area increased significantly ($3.2\pm0.6$ cm$^2$ vs $4.3\pm0.7$ cm$^2$, $p<0.00001$) (Figs. 7.8, 7.9 and 7.10) These data clearly demonstrate that artificially created double orifice valves follow a physiologic behaviour during exercise with a good valvular reserve in response to the increased cardiac output.

**Fig. 7.8** Response of mean
(**a**) and maximum (**b**) mitral
gradient to exercise after EE
repair

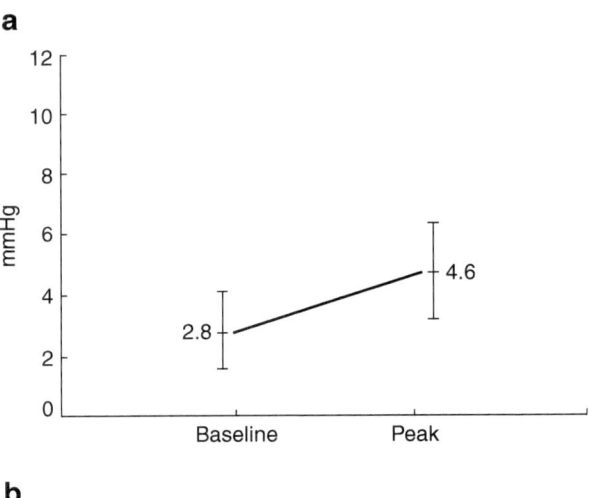

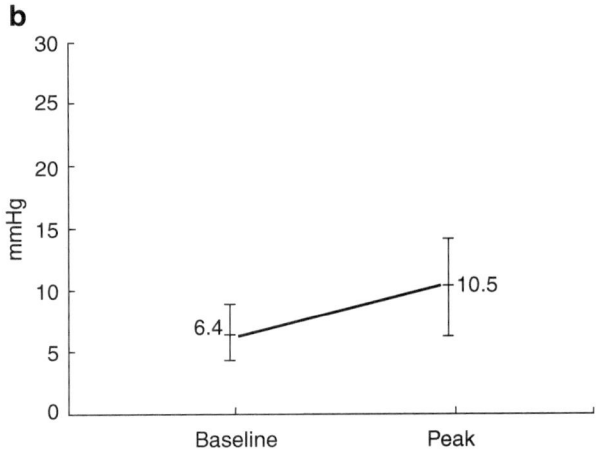

**Fig. 7.9** Exercise-induced
change in systolic
pulmonary artery pressure
after EE repair

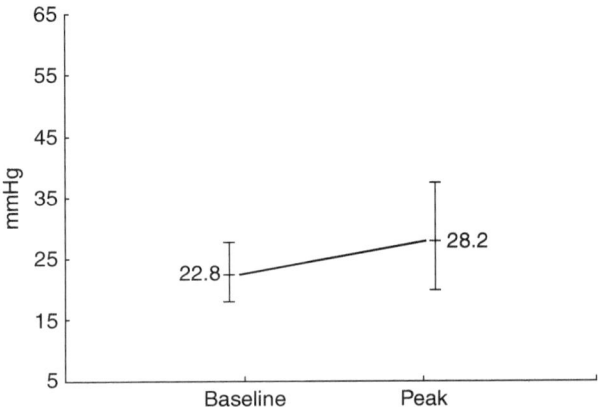

**Fig. 7.10** Exercise-induced change in planimetric mitral valve area after EE repair

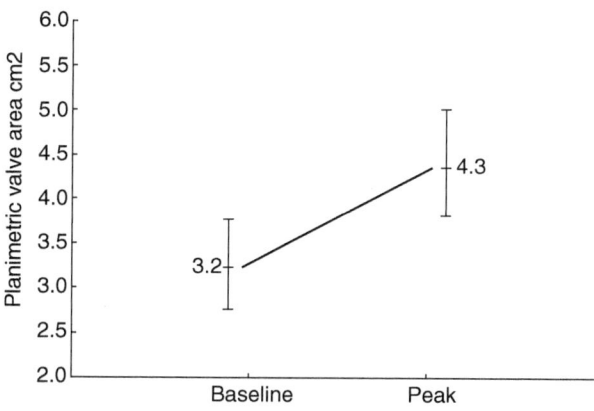

## Conclusions

Twenty years after its introduction, the EE technique remains an effective and versatile method to treat mitral regurgitation due to different etiologies and mechanisms. Simplicity, reliability and reproducibility are the main advantages of this method of repair. Indications and contraindications to the EE technique have been progressively refined over the years. As for any surgical technique, the only way to validate the EE approach is by means of standard outcome measures and analysis. The excellent long-term results which are now available confirm that, with appropriate patients' selection, the supposed drawbacks and risks of this technique are more theoretical than practical. Indeed, if properly applied, this "functional" rather than "anatomical" repair does not cause any significant restriction both at rest and during exercise and provides excellent efficacy and durability up to 20 years after the operation.

## References

1. Fucci C, Sandrelli L, Pardini A, et al. Improved results with mitral valve repair using new surgical techniques. Eur J Cardiothorac Surg. 1995;9:621–6.
2. Alfieri O, Maisano F, De Bonis M, et al. The double-orifice technique in mitral valve repair: a simple solution for complex problems. J Thorac Cardiovasc Surg. 2001;122:674–81.
3. Kuduvalli M, Ghotkar SV, Grayson AD, Fabri BM. Edge-to-edge technique for mitral valve repair: medium-term results with echocardiographic follow-up. Ann Thorac Surg. 2006;82: 1356–61.
4. Brinster DR, Unic D, D'Ambra MN, et al. Midterm results of the edge-to-edge technique for complex mitral valve repair. Ann Thorac Surg. 2006;81:1612–7.
5. Bhudia SK, McCarthy PM, Smedira NG, et al. Edge-to-edge (Alfieri) mitral repair: results in diverse clinical settings. Ann Thorac Surg. 2004;77:1598–606.
6. Kherani AR, Cheema FH, Casher J, et al. Edge-to-edge mitral valve repair: the Columbia Presbyterian experience. Ann Thorac Surg. 2004;78:73–6.
7. De Bonis M, Lapenna E, La Canna G, et al. Mitral valve repair for functional mitral regurgitation in end-stage dilated cardiomyopathy: the role of the "edge-to-edge" technique. Circulation. 2005;112(suppl I):I402–8.

8. De Bonis M, Lapenna E, Maisano F, Barili F, La Canna G, Buzzatti N, Pappalardo F, Calabrese M, Nisi T, Alfieri O. Long-term results (≤18 years) of the edge-to-edge mitral valve repair without annuloplasty in degenerative mitral regurgitation: implications for the percutaneous approach. Circulation. 2014;130(11 Suppl 1):S19–24.
9. Maisano F, Schreuder JJ, Oppizzi M, et al. The double-orifice technique as a standardized approach to treat mitral regurgitation due to severe myxomatous disease: surgical technique. Eur J Cardiothorac Surg. 2000;17:201–5.
10. De Bonis M, Lapenna E, Lorusso R, Buzzati N, Gelsomino S, Taramasso M, Vizzardi E, Alfieri O. Very long-term results (up to 17 years) with the double-orifice mitral valve repair combined with ring annuloplasty for degenerative mitral regurgitation. J Thorac Cardiovasc Surg. 2013;145(2):617.
11. Braunberger E, Deloche A, Berrei A, et al. Very long-term results (more than 20 years) of valve repair with Carpentier's techniques in nonrheumatic mitral valve insufficiency. Circulation. 2001;104(suppl I):I-8–11.
12. DiBardino DJ, ElBardissi AW, McClure RS, et al. Four decades of experience with mitral valve repair: analysis of differential indications, technical evolution, and long-term outcome. J Thorac Cardiovasc Surg. 2010;139:76–83.
13. Salvador L, Mirone S, Bianchini R, et al. A 20-year experience with mitral valve repair with artificial chordae in 608 patients. J Thorac Cardiovasc Surg. 2008;135:1280–7.
14. David TE, Armstrong S, McCrindle BW, Manlhiot C. Late outcomes of mitral valve repair for mitral regurgitation due to degenerative disease. Circulation. 2013;127(14):1485–92.
15. De Bonis M, Lapenna E, Taramasso M, La Canna G, Buzzatti N, Pappalardo F, Alfieri O. Very long-term durability of the edge-to-edge repair for isolated anterior mitral leaflet prolapse: up to 21 years of clinical and echocardiographic results. J Thorac Cardiovasc Surg. 2014;148(5):2027–32.
16. Gillinov AM, Cosgrove DM, Blackstone EH, Diaz R, Arnold JH, Lytle BW, et al. Durability of mitral valve repair for degenerative disease. J Thorac Cardiovasc Surg. 1998;116:734–43.
17. Suri RM, Schaff HV, Dearani JA, Sundt III TM, Daly RC, Mullany CJ, et al. Survival advantage and improved durability of mitral repair for leaflet prolapse subsets in the current era. Ann Thorac Surg. 2006;82:819–26.
18. Seeburger J, Borger MA, Doll N, Walther T, Passage J, Falk V, et al. Comparison of outcomes of minimally invasive mitral valve surgery for posterior, anterior and bileaflet prolapse. Eur J Cardiothorac Surg. 2009;36:532–8.
19. Castillo JG, Anyanwu AC, El-Eshmawi A, Adams DH. All anterior and bileaflet mitral valve prolapse are repairable in the modern era of reconstructive surgery. Eur J Cardiothorac Surg. 2014;45(1):139–45.
20. David TE, Armstrong S, Ivanov J. Chordal replacement with polytetrafluoroethylene sutures for mitral valve repair: a 25-year experience. J Thorac Cardiovasc Surg. 2013;145:1563–9.
21. Dreyfus G, Al Ayle N, Dubois C, de Lentdecker P. Long term results of mitral valve repair: posterior papillary muscle repositioning versus chordal shortening. Eur J Cardiothorac Surg. 1999;16:81–7.
22. De Bonis M, Lorusso R, Lapenna E, Kassem S, De Cicco G, Torracca L, et al. Similar long-term results of mitral valve repair for anterior compared with posterior leaflet prolapse. J Thorac Cardiovasc Surg. 2006;131:364–70.
23. Gillinov AM, Blackstone EH, Alaulaqi A, Sabik 3rd JF, Mihaljevic T, Svensson LG, et al. Outcomes after repair of the anterior mitral leaflet for degenerative disease. Ann Thorac Surg. 2008;86:708–17.
24. Mathieu P, Dagenais F, De Ibarra JIS, Baillot R. Surgical treatment of commissural prolapse: case report and review of the options. J Heart Valve Dis. 2004;13:142–4.
25. Aubert S, Barreda T, Acar C, Leprince P, Bonnet N, Ecochard R, Pavie A, Gandjbakhch I. Mitral valve repair for commissural prolapse: surgical techniques and long term results. Eur J Cardiothorac Surg. 2005;28:443–7.
26. Van Herwerden LA, Taams MA, Bos E. Repair of commissural prolapse by extended leaflet sliding. Ann Thorac Surg. 1994;57:387–90.
27. Gillinov AM, Shortt KG, Cosgrove III DM. Commissural closure for repair of mitral commissural prolapse. Ann Thorac Surg. 2005;80:1135–6.

28. Lapenna E, De Bonis M, Sorrentino F, La Canna G, Grimaldi A, Torracca L, Maisano F, Alfieri O. Commissural closure for the treatment of commissural mitral valve prolapse or flail. J Heart Valve Dis. 2008;17(3):261–6.
29. De Bonis M, Lapenna E, Taramasso M, Pozzoli A, La Canna G, Calabrese MC, Alfieri O. Is commissural closure associated with mitral annuloplasty a durable technique for the treatment of mitral regurgitation? A long-term (≤15 years) clinical and echocardiographic study. J Thorac Cardiovasc Surg. 2014;147(6):1900–6.
30. Joint Task Force on the Management of Valvular Heart Disease of the European Society of Cardiology (ESC); European Association for Cardio-Thoracic Surgery (EACTS), Vahanian A, Alfieri O, Andreotti F, Antunes MJ, Barón-Esquivias G, Baumgartner H, Borger MA, Carrel TP, De Bonis M, Evangelista A, Falk V, Iung B, Lancellotti P, Pierard L, Price S, Schäfers HJ, Schuler G, Stepinska J, Swedberg K, Takkenberg J, Von Oppell UO, Windecker S, Zamorano JL, Zembala M. Guidelines on the management of valvular heart disease (version 2012). Eur Heart J. 2012;33:2451–96.
31. Umana JP, Salehizadeh BS, DeRose JJ, Nahar T, Lotvin A, Homma S, et al. "Bow-tie" mitral valve repair: an adjuvant technique for ischemic mitral regurgitation. Ann Thorac Surg. 1998;66:1640–6.
32. Kinnaird TD, Munt BI, Ignaszewski AP, Abel JG, Thompson CR. Edge-to-edge repair for functional mitral regurgitation: an echocardiographic study of the hemodynamic consequences. J Heart Valve Dis. 2003;12:280–6.
33. De Bonis M, Lapenna E, Verzini A, La Canna G, Grimaldi A, Torracca L, et al. Recurrence of mitral regurgitation parallels the absence of left ventricular reverse remodeling after mitral repair in advanced dilated cardiomyopathy. Ann Thorac Surg. 2008;85(3):932–9.
34. Hung J, Papakostas L, Tahta SA, Hardy BG, Bollen BA, Duran CM, et al. Mechanism of recurrent ischemic mitral regurgitation after annuloplasty: continued LV remodeling as a moving target. Circulation. 2004;110:II85–90.
35. Freeman WK, Schaff HV, Khandheria BK, et al. Intraoperative evaluation of mitral valve regurgitation and repair by transesophageal echocardiography: incidence and significance of systolic anterior motion. J Am Coll Cardiol. 1992;20:599–609.
36. Mascagni R, Al Attar N, Lamarra M, et al. Edge-to-edge technique to treat post-mitral valve repair systolic anterior motion and left ventricular outflow tract obstruction. Ann Thorac Surg. 2005;79:471–3.
37. Myers PO, Khalpey Z, Maloney AM, et al. Edge-to-edge repair for prevention and treatment of mitral valve systolic anterior motion. J Thorac Cardiovasc Surg. J Thorac Cardiovasc Surg. 2013;146(4):836–40.
38. Wan CK, Dearani JA, Sundt 3rd TM, et al. What is the best surgical treatment for obstructive hypertrophic cardiomyopathy and degenerative mitral regurgitation? Ann Thorac Surg. 2009;88(3):727–31.
39. Agricola E, Oppizzi M, Maisano F, Bove T, De Bonis M, Toracca L, Alfieri O. Detection of mechanisms of immediate failure by transesophageal echocardiography in quadrangular resection mitral valve repair technique for severe mitral regurgitation. Am J Cardiol. 2003;91:175–9, 599–609.
40. Gatti G, Cardu G, Trane R, Pugliese P. The edge-to-edge technique as a trick to rescue an imperfect mitral valve repair. Eur J Cardiothorac Surg. 2002;22:817–20.
41. De Bonis M, Lapenna E, Buzzatti N, Taramasso M, Calabrese MC, Nisi T, Pappalardo F, Alfieri O. Can the edge-to-edge technique provide durable results when used to rescue patients with suboptimal conventional mitral repair? Eur J Cardiothorac Surg. 2013;43(6):e173–9.
42. Agricola E, Maisano F, Oppizzi M, et al. Mitral valve reserve in double-orifice technique: an exercise echocardiographic study. J Heart Valve Dis. 2002;11(5):637–43.
43. Frapier JM, Sportouch C, Rauzy V, et al. Mitral valve repair by Alfieri's technique does not limit exercise tolerance more than Carpentier's correction. Eur J Cardiothorac Surg. 2006;29:1020–5.

# Edge-to-Edge Technique for Mitral Regurgitation Associated with Hypertrophic Cardiomyopathy

8

Jean-François Obadia

## 8.1 Introduction

Many surgical techniques have been described to treat mitral regurgitation (MR) associated with hypertrophic cardiomyopathy (HCM) (sometimes contradictory: i.e., both shortening [1] and elongation [2] of the anterior leaflet), which probably illustrates confusion in the interpretation of the disease. Mitral regurgitation due to HCM is mainly functional (secondary) as a consequence of systolic anterior motion (SAM) of the anterior leaflet. Two dysfunction mechanisms account for SAM (Fig. 8.1): a pulling mechanism due to a Venturi effect in the outflow tract, and a pushing effect due to the force of flow exerted on the distal part of the anterior leaflet. Moreover, an organic MR mechanism is also possible, due to a too long anterior leaflet or abnormal anatomy or position of the papillary muscles. Taken together, these mechanisms are responsible for severe MR in more than 30 % of cases of HCM in surgical series [3].

According to the guidelines [4, 5] the basis of treatment for HCM consists in removing the hypertrophic septum (Morrow principle), leading to excellent and reproducible surgical results reported by experienced teams [6], our own policy is to stick to this principle. Nevertheless, in case of severe MR, we add an edge-to-edge stitch, which is very helpful in order to secure correction of both the obstruction and the MR.

J.-F. Obadia
Service de Chirurgie Cardiothoracique et Transplantation, Hôpital Cardiothoracique Louis Pradel, Lyon-Bron, France

Laboratoire de Physiologie Lyon Nord, UCBL1, INSERM, U 886 "Cardioprotection", Lyon, France
e-mail: jean-francois.obadia@chu-lyon.fr

© Springer International Publishing Switzerland 2015
O. Alfieri et al. (eds.), *Edge-to-Edge Mitral Repair: From a Surgical to a Percutaneous Approach*, DOI 10.1007/978-3-319-19893-4_8

**Fig. 8.1** Two dysfunction mechanisms explain SAM: a pulling mechanism (*blue arrow*) due to a Venturi effect in the outflow tract, and a pushing effect (*green arrow*) due to the direct force of the flow exerted on the distal part of the anterior leaflet

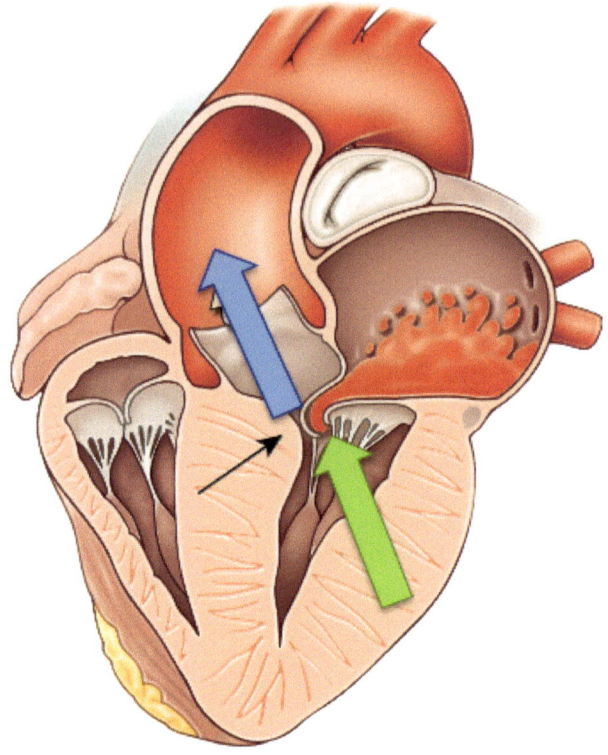

## 8.2    Surgical Technique

The procedure begins and finishes with transesophageal echography (TEE) assessment, to describe the abnormal anatomy to correct (Fig. 8.2) and then to assess of the quality of the result.

- The procedure is performed on bypass between a single double-stage venous cannula and an aortic cannula with cardiologic cardiac arrest. The aorta is opened transversally and the whole procedure is performed through the aortic orifice without any additional incision, and in particular without any direct opening of the left atrium.
- The first step starts with resection of the hypertrophic septum according to a modified Morrow procedure: i.e., broad resection starting 2 mm below the nadir of the right cusp (remote from the conduction pathway), going below the right-left commissure and finishing 2 mm below the nadir of the left cusp. Resection is then extended deeply into the left ventricle (LV), down to the two papillary muscles. Sometimes big papillary muscles have to be reduced and/or detached from the LV wall. Any additional papillary muscles with direct connection to the leaflets have to be sectioned and entirely resected.

**Fig. 8.2** In this echographic systolic view, aortic valve open (*Ao*), obstruction is partly due to a huge bulging septum (*S*), SAM and a muscular attachment between anterior leaflet and septum (*arrow*)

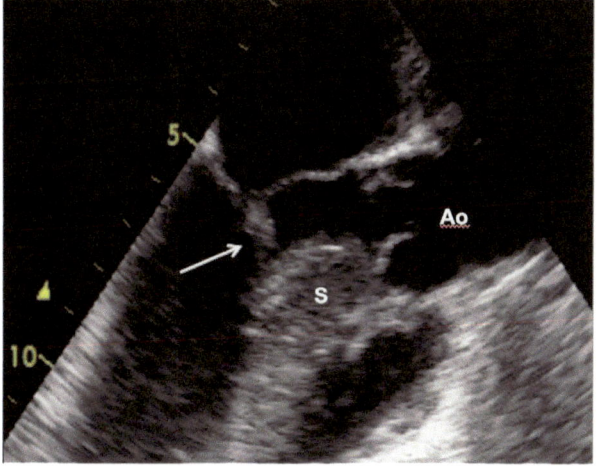

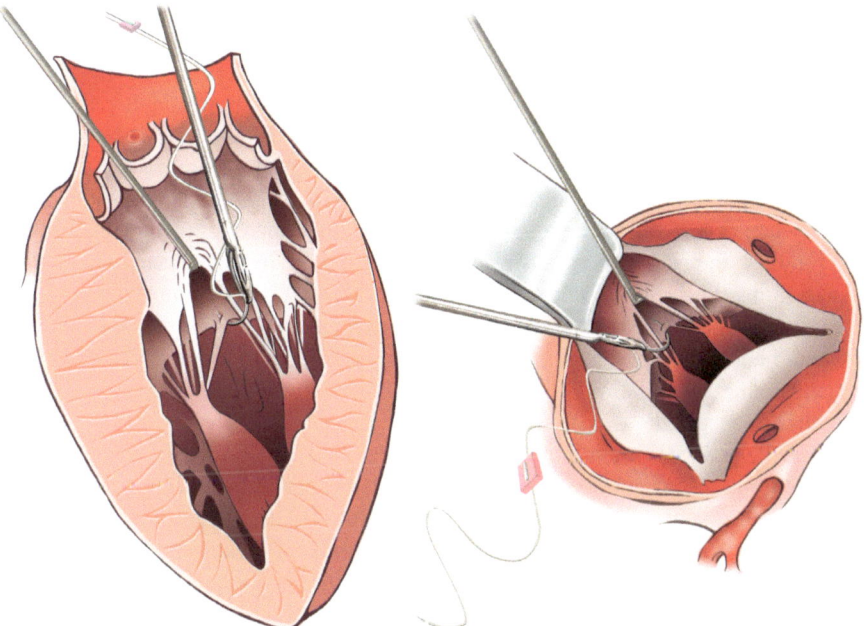

**Figs. 8.3 and 8.4** The pledgeted (piece of autologous pericardium) edge-to-edge U suture is placed in the central part of the leaflets (A2 and P2) on either side

- The second step consists in edge-to-edge U suture, reinforced by 2 autologous pericardial pledgets (Figs. 8.3 and 8.4). The pericardial pledgets are easily taken out in situ. Through the aortic orifice, a hook pulls back the anterior leaflet, giving a direct view of the free edge of the posterior leaflet (Fig. 8.5). P2 and A2 are easily located, being situated between the chordae on either side.

**Fig. 8.5** Operative view of edge-to-edge suture positioning after an extended Morrow procedure, which provides good exposure of the sub-valvular apparatus

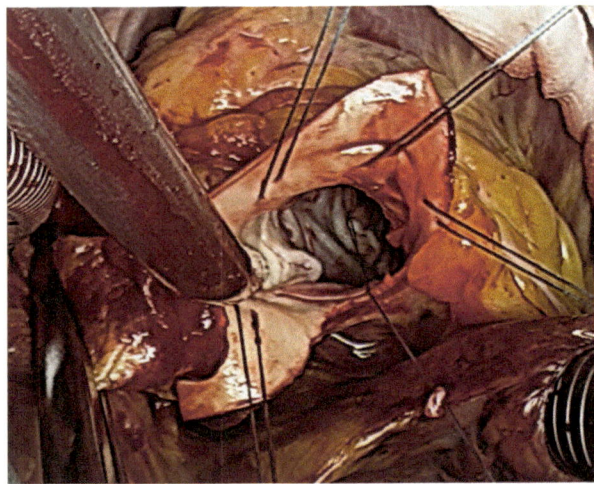

## 8.3    Results

For pure secondary MR, the original and, even more, the enlarged Morrow resection technique is usually enough to treat both the direct obstruction due to the enlarged septum and the indirect obstruction due to the SAM. In case of huge SAM, particularly when associated with an abnormal sub-valvular apparatus requiring additional techniques, the risk is to impair mitral valve function. In such cases, we decided to add a transaortic edge-to-edge suture to secure the MR correction.

Ten patients were operated on with this procedure. The second patient showed detachment of the edge-to-edge suture on day 3, leading to grade 2 MR due to a tear in the leaflet (no SAM). Thereafter, from patients 3–10, we added pericardial patches to secure the A2-P2 suture.

The 10 patients (including patient 2) had uneventful follow-up with good clinical outcome. Mean intra-ventricular gradient decreased from 76 to 6 mmHg. MR was absent or only trivial in the 9 patients with efficient edge-to-edge technique. Mean trans-mitral valvular gradient was 3 mmHg. All patients underwent stress echo at 6 months, with no significant gradient either inside the ventricle or through the mitral valve.

### Conclusion
The enlarged Morrow procedure remains the gold standard and main step of any surgery for HCM. In case of severe MR, particularly when associated with abnormal sub-valvular apparatus anatomy requiring direct correction, adding an edge-to-edge suture is helpful to secure coaptation between the two leaflets. In complex MR mechanisms, this technique avoids associating a more questionable direct procedure on the mitral valve, requiring left atrium opening or, even worse, valve replacement, which should be exceptional.

# References

1. Swistel DG, Balaram SK. Surgical myectomy for hypertrophic cardiomyopathy in the 21st century, the evolution of the "RPR" repair: resection, plication, and release. Prog Cardiovasc Dis. 2012;54:498–502.
2. Van der Lee C, ten Cate FJ, Geleijnse ML, et al. Percutaneous versus surgical treatment for patients with hypertrophic obstructive cardiomyopathy and enlarged anterior mitral valve leaflets. Circulation. 2005;112:482–8.
3. Mohr R, Schaff HV, Danielson GK, et al. The outcome of surgical treatment of hypertrophic obstructive cardiomyopathy. Experience over 15 years. J Thorac Cardiovasc Surg. 1989;97: 666–74.
4. Gersh BJ, Maron BJ, Bonow RO, et al. 2011 ACCF/AHA guideline for the diagnosis and treatment of hypertrophic cardiomyopathy: a report of the American College of Cardiology Foundation/American Heart Association Task Force on Practice Guidelines. Circulation. 2011;124:e783–831.
5. Elliott PM, Anastasakis A, Borger MA, et al. ESC Guidelines on diagnosis and management of hypertrophic cardiomyopathy. Eur Heart J. 2014. doi:10.1093/eurheartj/ehu284.
6. Maron BJ. Surgical myectomy remains the primary treatment option for severely symptomatic patients with obstructive hypertrophic cardiomyopathy. Circulation. 2007;116:196–206.

# Mitral Stenosis After Edge-to-Edge Repair: Is It an Issue?

9

### Giovanna Di Giannuario and Giovanni La Canna

## 9.1   Introduction

The edge-to-edge (EE) repair, also known as "Alfieri's stitch" is a reproducible and effective technique to restore mitral valve (MV) competence. In the past decade the EE repair has played an established role in the MV surgical repair armamentarium [1–3]. When this technique is applied in the central part of the anterior and posterior MV leaflets, two orifices are created and the effective MV area is significantly reduced.

The so called "double-orifice mitral valve" (DOMV) is an uncommon congenital anomaly, with an incidence of 0.05 % in the general population. It was first described by Greenfield in 1876 and it is often associated with other congenital defects. The hemodynamic effects of a DOMV vary from normally functioning valves to significant mitral regurgitation (MR) or mitral stenosis (MS). In one of the largest series in the literature (46 children) with DOMV, MR was the most frequent finding (43 %), whereas MS prevalence was 13 %, and a combination of MS and insufficiency was found in 6.5 % of patients [4–9].

As in the case of the congenital defect, the possible negative outcome of the EE surgical technique is more frequently represented by MR than MS.

## 9.2   Computational Model Analysis

Clinical experience, 3D-computational models and in vitro studies have demonstrated that the hemodynamic performance of a double orifice valve is similar to that of a single orifice one with the same total effective orifice area [10, 11].

G. Di Giannuario (✉) • G. La Canna
Department of Cardiac Surgery, IRCCS San Raffaele University Hospital,
Via Olgettina, 60, Milan 20100, Italy
e-mail: gdigiannuario@gmail.com

© Springer International Publishing Switzerland 2015
O. Alfieri et al. (eds.), *Edge-to-Edge Mitral Repair: From a Surgical
to a Percutaneous Approach*, DOI 10.1007/978-3-319-19893-4_9

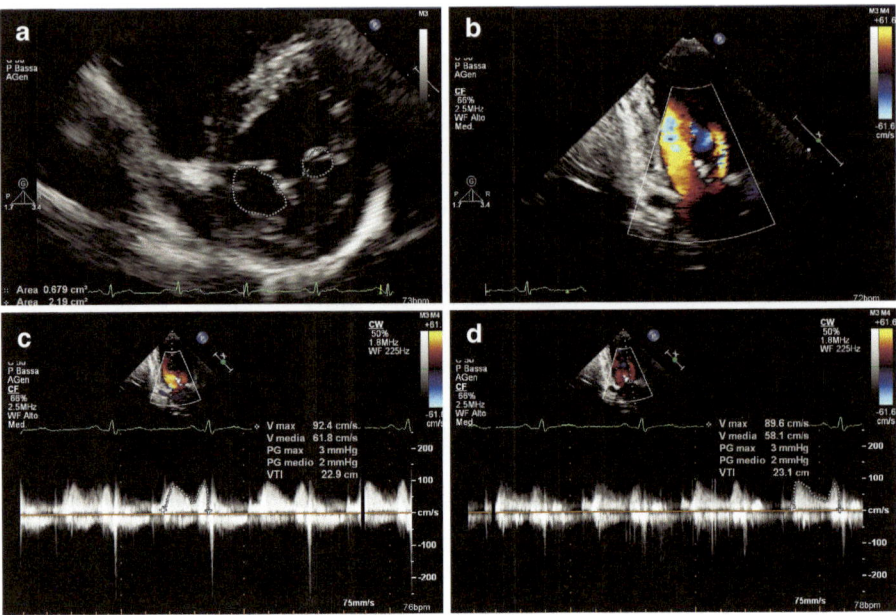

**Fig. 9.1** Echocardiographic Color Doppler assessment in vivo of trans-mitral gradient after an asymmetrical EE repair: (**a**) Effective orifice area in asymmetric double orifice; (**b**) Color Doppler imaging of the double inflow; (**c**) Echo-Doppler with peak and mean gradient values in the postero-medial orifice (the larger one, 2 cm² area); (**d**) Echo-Doppler with peak and mean gradient values probed in the antero-lateral orifice, the smaller one. The trans-mitral gradient values are the same according to the 3D computational study findings

In particular, flow velocity and pressure drop through each orifice are similar to those registered in a single orifice valve with the same total area. Moreover, flow velocity and pressure drop are exactly the same in the two orifices, even when they have different sizes (asymmetrical EE). Indeed the flow velocity is mainly related to the atrio-ventricular decay, regardless of the double orifice-shape of the MV inflow [5] (see Chap. 2, Figs. 2.2 and 2.3). Those findings also justify the applicability of the echo-Doppler examination to assess the results of the surgical EE repair. During echo-color Doppler echocardiography the flow through the valve can be probed in any of the two orifices, even if they have different sizes, providing data on the overall valve performance (flow velocity, pressure gradient, functional valve area) (Fig. 9.1).

## 9.3    Determinants of the Risk of MV Stenosis After EE Repair

To assess the occurrence of stenosis post EE repair, we can use the same criteria adopted in case of a native MV. Typical indexes like valve area, mean gradient and pulmonary pressure can be integrated to define the presence and severity of MV stenosis (Table 9.1).

**Table 9.1**  Recommendations for mitral stenosis severity, at heart rates between 60 and 80 bpm and in sinus rhythm

|  | Mild | Moderate | Severe |
|---|---|---|---|
| *Specific finding* | | | |
| Valve area (cm²) | >1.5 | 1–1.5 | <1 |
| *Supportive findings* | | | |
| Mean gradient (mmHg) | <5 | 5–10 | >10 |
| Pulmonary artery pressure | <30 | 30–50 | >50 |

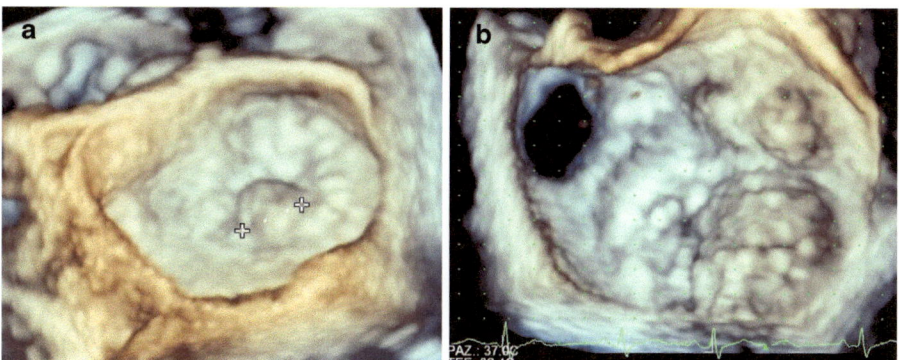

**Fig. 9.2**  Example of intercommissural extension of prolapse. (**a**) Ideal lesion with an extension suitable for the EE technique. (**b**) Complex lesion, bileaflets prolapse with a wide intercommissural extension at higher risk of post-repair EE stenosis

The risk of postoperative stenosis is higher in case of large intercommisural extension of the MV lesions and in presence of a small native valve area (Fig. 9.2). Careful attention needs to be paid to the length of the EE suture and to the size of the ring in order to maintain an acceptable residual anatomical area which should be larger than 2.5 cm² [10, 11] (Fig. 9.3).

A major risk of stenosis after EE repair is therefore present in presence of:

1. Small native valve area
2. Large intercommisural width of the prolapsing lesion
3. Large intercommissural extension of the surgical suture
4. Restrictive annuloplasty

The experience of the surgical team and the selection of the patient play a key role in preventing the occurrence of this complication. In a group of patients with degenerative MR and long-term (≤18 years) echocardiographic follow-up after EE repair, reported by our Institution, the incidence of postoperative MS was 0.6 % [12, 13].

This issue has been investigated by several studies during the first years after the introduction of the EE technique. Exercise stress echocardiography has been used to establish the clinical meaning of the effective reduction of the preoperative MV orifice area.

**Fig. 9.3** Computational 3D model demonstrated the influence of the total orifice area on the pressure gradients at 11 l/min. $\Delta p_{max}$: maximum pressure gradient across the valve; $\Delta p_{Bernoulli}$: pressure gradient calculated with the simplified Bernoulli formula ($4\,V^2_{max}$) (Reproduced with permission from [11])

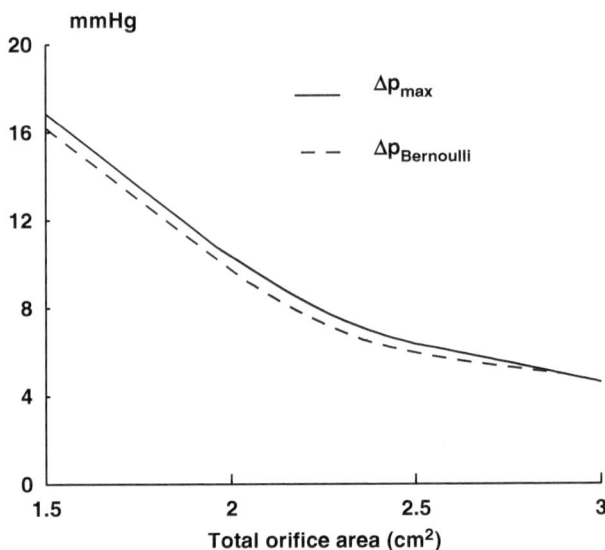

In particular, Frapier et al. compared the pathophysiology of the MV after double-orifice repair (25 pts, group A) or conventional Carpentier's repair (29 pts, group C). A control group of ten healthy subjects was also included [14]. Rest/exercise echocardiography and cardiorespiratory testing with maximal oxygen uptake were performed in all patients: baseline MV area was significantly larger in group C compared to group A (2.9 cm$^2$ vs. 2.5 cm$^2$, $p=0.0018$). However, despite the higher MV area reduction, the EE technique did not increase the transvalvular gradients more than the traditional Carpentier's repair: the mean mitral gradients at rest were 3.8 mmHg in the EE group and 3.3 mmHg in the traditional technique.

The maximum oxygen uptake (VO$_2$ max) was comparable between the two surgical groups and the normal subjects. These data show that the EE repair, despite the higher reduction of the MV area at rest, does not induce higher transvalvular gradients at rest or under exercise than conventional repairs and provides the same effectiveness in reducing MR as well as the same exercise tolerance [14]. In our Institution we have been measuring gradients at rest across the MV following EE repair since the beginning. MS was exceptionally observed immediately after surgery and never at follow-up. In addition, we performed exercise echocardiography (10 W/min) in 30 patients previously submitted to MV repair. At the peak of the stress, heart rate, systolic blood pressure and stroke volume significantly increased, confirming a physiological behavior of the MV. The mean MV gradient ($2.8\pm1.3$ mmHg vs. $4.6\pm1.9$ mmHg, $p<0.00001$), the maximum MV gradient ($6.4\pm2.8$ mmHg vs. $10.5\pm4.6$ mmHg, $p<0.00002$) and the systolic pulmonary artery pressure ($22.8\pm6.1$ mmHg vs. $28.2\pm9.9$ mmHg, $p<0.001$) increased, but not to pathological levels. The planimetric valve area increased significantly ($3.2\pm0.6$ cm$^2$ vs $4.3\pm0.7$ cm$^2$, $p<0.00001$) [18].

These results have further proved that functional MS does not develop after the EE repair neither at rest nor under exercise.

## 9.4 How to Evaluate Post-EE Repair MS

Echocardiographic evaluation and grading of MS in a native valve is usually based on an integrated approach, using different anatomical and Doppler quantitative measures (Table 9.2). The principal methods to evaluate MS are: planimetric orifice area, pressure half time (PHT), deceleration time, continuity equation, sPAP (systolic pulmonary artery pressure), trans-mitral gradient, pulmonary vein flow pattern, isovolumetric relaxation time (IVRT), proximal isovelocity surface area (PISA). A perfect comprehensive measure of significant MS after repair does not exist. The Doppler methods (PHT, continuity equation, PISA) are highly influenced by blood flow, heart rate and compliance of the left ventricle and left atrium. The peak and mean pressure gradients are dependent on transvalvular flow and diastolic filling period and will vary greatly with changes in heart rate. Atrial fibrillation with an irregular heart rate poses additional problems, and changes in the diastolic filling time may induce a dramatic variation in the mean transvalvular gradient [22–24, 29, 30].

### 9.4.1 Intraoperative Anatomic Determination of the Severity of MS

In order to establish the acute onset of MS after the EE technique, it is mandatory to perform transesophageal echocardiography (TOE) in the operating room right after weaning from cardiopulmonary bypass, thus evaluating the two-dimensional (2D) planimetry of the MV and the total area with the sum of the two orifices.

Planimetry is the direct measurement of the double orifice area, which may be visualized in the transgastric short axis view, where the image is frozen in early diastole which corresponds to maximal valve opening. The limitation of the 2D planimetry of the double orifice is that, sometimes, the area of the two orifices is not visible on the same plane, leading to possible underestimation of the total orifice area. This problem is solved by the new 3D echocardiography technology with zoom acquisition and Qlab analysis.

In case of poor image quality of the transesophageal transgastric windows, it is possible to obtain an epicardial evaluation of the double orifice mitral inflow.

The use of 3D echocardiography and the assessment of the double orifice area through 3D Quantitative Mitral Valve software analysis is becoming the gold standard for the evaluation of a possible MS post surgical repair (Figs. 9.4 and 9.5).

### 9.4.2 Intraoperative Doppler Echocardiographic Determination of the MS Severity

PHT Doppler evaluation, deceleration time, PISA and standard continuity equation are the established methods of MV stenosis grading in native valves and in rest conditions. The limitations of those methods, however, depend on the fact that they

**Table 9.2** Methods for the evaluation and grading of mitral valve stenosis in native valves

| Measurement | Unit | Formula/method | Concept | Advantage | Disadvantage |
|---|---|---|---|---|---|
| Valve area Planimetry 2D/3D | cm$^2$ | 2D/3D echo Tracing of the mitral orifice | Direct measurement of anatomic MVA | Accuracy Independence from other factors | Experienced required Not always feasible (poor acoustic window, severe valve calcification) |
| PHT (pressure half Time) | cm$^2$ | 220/T1/2 | Rate of decrease of trans-mitral flow is inversely proportional to MVA | Easy to obtain | Dependence on other factors (AR, LA compliance, LV compliance and function, etc.) |
| Continuity Equation | cm$^2$ | MVA$=(D^2/4)$ (VTI aortic/VTI mitral) | Volume flows through aorta and mitral orifices are equal | Independence of flow condition | Multiple measurements (sources of errors) and not valid in presence of significant AR and MR |
| IVRT | cm | Shortening in severe MS | Isovolumic relaxation time | Independence of flow condition | Influenced by left ventricle relaxation |
| PISA | cm$^2$ | MVA$=\{(2pr^2 \times v_a)/v_{peak}) \times (\alpha/180°)\}$ | Proximal isovolumetric Surface area | Independence of flow condition | Technically difficult |
| Mean gradient | mmHg | $\Delta P=\Sigma\ 4\ V^2/N$ | Pressure gradient obtained by velocity using modified Bernoulli equation | Easy to obtain | Dependent on flow condition and heart rate |
| Systolic pulmonary artery pressure | mmHg | sPAP$=4V^2_{tricuspid}$ $_+$ RA pressure | Addition of RA pressure an maximum gradient between RA-RV | Obtained in most patients | No estimation of pulmonary vascular resistance |
| Pulmonary vein pattern | Wave pattern | PVs/PVs+PVd | Pulsed Doppler | Very simple with TEE | Difficult transthoracic evaluation Influenced by LV function |

Adapted and modified from the AHA/ACC 2014 guidelines for heart valve disease

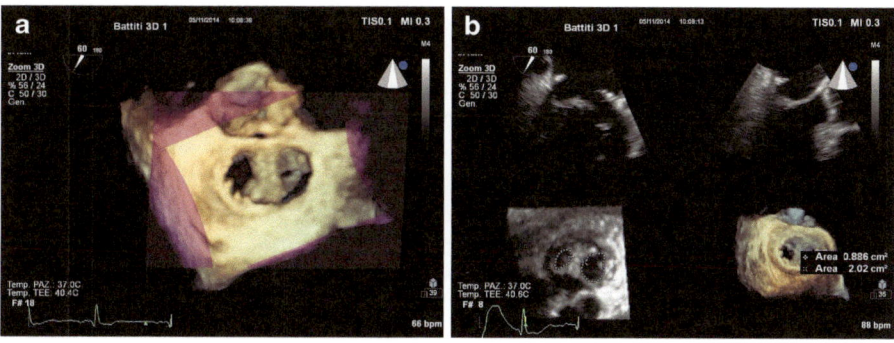

**Fig. 9.4** 3D zoom view of post-repair double orifice mitral valve (**a**), multiplanar analysis with Q Lab Philips system (**b**) with effective orifice area quantification

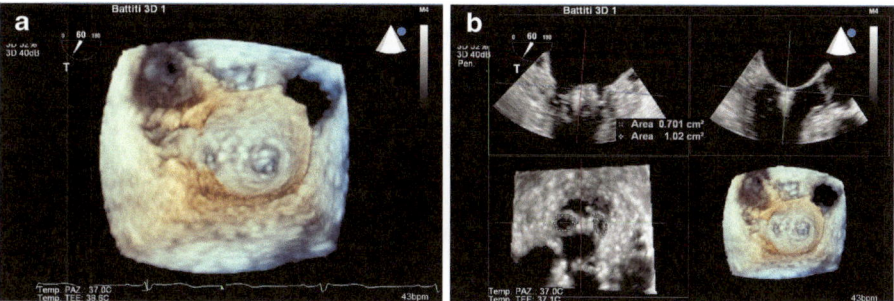

**Fig. 9.5** Post procedural result of two mitraclips implantation with 3D zoom evaluation of the double-orifice area

are influenced by flow condition, aortic valve regurgitation, atrio-ventricular compliance, heart rate and technical acquisition issues.

In the intraoperative setting they are not reliable tools, since they are influenced by many variables: cardiac output (CO), loading conditions (central venous pressure, CVP), systemic vascular resistance, heart rate (HR), heart rhythm, pacemaker stimulation, anemic status, hemodynamic conditions in general anesthesia (vasodilatation) and inotropic drugs. A recent study investigated the role of the trans-mitral gradients in the intraoperative evaluation of MV repair and identified a mean gradient ≥7 mmHg and a peak gradient >17 mmHg as pathological results, requiring MV replacement for acute iatrogenic MS [28].

The intraoperative factors previously mentioned (HR, CO, CVP, drugs, vascular resistance, catecholamine release, etc.) affect peak and mean gradients. For this reasons, we believe that 2D or 3D planimetry with systolic pulmonary artery pressure (sPAP) estimation and pulsed Doppler pulmonary vein pattern are the best echocardiographic indexes for the evaluation of MS in the intraoperative setting.

### 9.4.3 Postoperative Evaluation of MS

In the early postoperative period the patients often show anemia, arrhythmias and hypotension. The assessment of a possible MS has to be performed once all those confounding factors have been controlled. At mid/long-term follow-up, patients submitted to the EE repair should undergo a complete multiparametric transthoracic echocardiography with repeated measurements of trans-mitral peak and mean gradients, total double orifice area, left ventricular systolic function (ejection fraction), left atrium volume and pulmonary artery pressure. All those values should be compared with previous evaluations.

## 9.5 Management and Treatment of Post EE Repair MS

In the event of significant stenosis post-EE repair, if the patient is symptomatic, it is necessary to measure the effective total area of the two orifices and to assess the mean gradient and the sPAP. A total double-orifice valve area less than 1 cm$^2$ associated with a mean gradient greater than 10 mmHg and a high systolic pulmonary pressure (>50 mmHg) indicates significant MS requiring prosthetic MV replacement.

In asymptomatic patients with post-repair severe MS and in symptomatic patients with post-repair moderate stenosis (mean gradient 6–8 mmHg) the first step is represented by medical therapy, usually with beta-blockers that decrease the heart rate and increase the diastolic filling time. Then a new transesophageal (TOE) examination (possibly with 3D acquisition) should be performed to evaluate the effective double-orifice area planimetry. Since trans-mitral gradient and systolic pulmonary arterial pressure at rest often do not reflect the actual severity of MS, stress echocardiography can be particularly useful to assess valve function and its hemodynamic consequences, particularly in asymptomatic patients and in those with discordant Doppler findings at rest. Indeed some patients with only moderate planimetric stenosis at rest may show exercise-induced pulmonary hypertension and exertional dyspnea.

According to the current guidelines, in presence of a native MV, an increase in the systolic pulmonary pressure (>60 mmHg), the presence of left ventricular maladaptation, or an increase in the trans-mitral mean gradient > 15 mmHg during exercise (in the absence of high blood pressure, significant coronary disease or other valve disease) indicate the need of valve intervention [25]. Obviously, after an EE repair, the results of the exercise test must be correlated to the planimetric pathological reduction of the double orifice area. In recent studies, patients submitted to different types of MV repair (other than EE) with ring annuloplasty were investigated by stress echocardiography. The residual MV area was identified as one of the major independent predictors of exercise capacity, cardiac hemodynamic and quality of life [26, 27].

## 9.6    Evaluation of MV After the MitraClip Procedure

In the current era of percutaneous EE repair with the MitraClip system, 2D and 3D echocardiography plays a central role during the procedure and in the final evaluation of residual regurgitation, MV area and possible stenosis. The MitraClip system creates the same double orifice configuration of the MV generated by the surgical procedure and has become an important therapeutic option in patients with significant comorbidities and high surgical risk [21]. The role of echocardiography is crucial to select the patient, guide the procedure and assess the result. One of the most important criteria in selecting MitraClip candidates is the presence of a basal MV area $\geq 4$ cm$^2$ [20]. The aim in performing the percutaneous EE repair is to have the maximal MR reduction with the smallest number of clips implanted. This is particularly important in the setting of functional MR, in which the baseline area is smaller than in degenerative disease, and the left ventricular and atrial pressure are both significantly increased due to severe systo-diastolic cardiac dysfunction.

---

**Conclusions**

In conclusion, if the EE technique is correctly applied, a postoperative functional MS does not occur and a real anatomical stenosis is a very rare event. The most important determinants of post-repair mitral valve stenosis are the selection of the patient and the expertise of the surgical team. According to computational models, it is important to maintain a residual area larger than 2.5 cm$^2$ in normal size patients. All the parameters and derived calculations for the assessment of significant MS described in the literature have advantages and drawbacks, especially in the operating room just after weaning from the extracorporeal circulation. Therefore, the effective total orifice traced by 3D echocardiography is becoming the gold standard for the diagnosis of post-repair MS.

---

## References

1. Fedak PWM, McCarthy PM, Bonow RO. Evolving concepts and technologies in mitral valve repair. Circulation. 2008;117:963–74.
2. Maisano F, Schreuder JJ, Oppizzi M, Fiorani B, Fino C, Alfieri O. The double-orifice technique as a standardized approach to treat mitral regurgitation due to severe myxomatous disease: surgical technique. Eur J Cardiothorac Surg. 2000;17:201–5.
3. De Bonis M, Alfieri O. The edge-to-edge technique for mitral valve repair. HSR Proc Intensive Care Cardiovasc Anesth. 2010;2(1):7–17.
4. Takeshita K, Inden Y, Murohara T. Coincidental finding of isolated congenital double-orifice mitral valve in two adult patients. Eur J Echocardiogr. 2011;12(3), E26.
5. Patted SV, Halkati PC, Ambar SS, Sattur AG. Successful treatment of double-orifice mitral stenosis with percutaneous balloon mitral commissurotomy. Case Rep Cardiol. 2012;2012:315175.
6. Trowitzsch E, Bano-Rodrigo A, Burger BM, Colan SD, Sanders SP. Two-dimensional echocardiographic findings in double orifice mitral valve. J Am Coll Cardiol. 1985;6(2):383–7.
7. Allen HD, Gutgesell HP, Clark EB, Driscoll DJ. Moss and Adams' heart disease in infants, children, and adolescents: including the fetus and young adult. Lippincott Williams & Wilkins 7th ed. 2008.

8. Westendorp IC, de Bruin-Bon HA, Hrudova J. Double orifice mitral valve; a coincidental find-ing. Eur J Echocardiogr. 2006;7(6):463–4.
9. Zalzstein E, Hamilton R, Zucker N, et al. Presentation, natural history, and outcome in children and adolescents with double orifice mitral valve. Am J Cardiol. 2004;93:1067–9.
10. Votta E, Maisano F, Soncini M, Redaelli A, Montevecchi FM, Alfieri O. 3-D computational analysis of the stress distribution on the leaflets after edge-to-edge repair of mitral regurgita-tion. J Heart Valve Dis. 2002;11:810–22.
11. Maisano F, Redaelli A, Pennati G, et al. The hemodynamic effects of double-orifice valve repair for mitral regurgitation: a 3D computational model. Eur J Cardiothorac Surg. 1999;15:419–25.
12. De Bonis M, Lapenna E, Lorusso R, Buzzatti N, Gelsomino S, Taramasso M, Vizzardi E, Alfieri O. Very long-term results (up to 17 years) with the double-orifice mitral valve repair combined with ring annuloplasty for degenerative mitral regurgitation. J Thorac Cardiovasc Surg. 2012;144:1019–24.
13. De Bonis M, Lapenna E, Maisano F, Barili F, La Canna G, Buzzatti N, Pappalardo F, Calabrese M, Nisi T, Alfieri O. Long-term results (≤18 years) of the edge-to-edge mitral valve repair without annuloplasty in degenerative mitral regurgitation: implications for the percutaneous approach. Circulation. 2014;130(11 Suppl 1):S19–24.
14. Frapier JM, Sportouch C, Rauzy V, et al. Mitral valve repair by Alfieri's technique does not limit exercise tolerance more than Carpentier's correction. Eur J Cardiothorac Surg. 2006; 29:1020–5.
15. Bonser DRS, Pagano D, Laverich A. Mitral valve surgery book. Chapter 8. Book Springer 2011. p. 77–84.
16. Maisano F, Torracca L, Oppizzi M, Stefano PL, D'Addario G, La Canna G, et al. The edge-to-edge technique: a simplified method to correct mitral insufficiency. Eur J Cardiothorac Surg. 1998;13:240–5.
17. Maisano F, Caldarola A, Blasio A, De Bonis M, La Canna G, Alfieri O. Midterm results of edge-to-edge mitral valve repair without annuloplasty. J Thorac Cardiovasc Surg. 2003;126(6):1987–97.
18. Agricola E, Maisano F, Oppizzi M, La Canna G, Alfieri O. Mitral valve reserve in double-orifice technique: an exercise echocardiographic study. J Heart Valve Dis. 2002;11:637–43.
19. Fedak PWM, McCarthy PM, Patrick M, Bonow RO. Evolving concepts and technologies in Mitral Valve Repair Circulation. 2008;117(7):963–74.
20. Feldman SK, Rinaldi M, Fail P, Hermiller J, Smalling R, Whitlow PL, et al. Percutaneous mitral repair with the MitraClip system: safety and midterm durability in the initial EVEREST (Endovascular Valve Edge-to-Edge Repair Study) cohort. J Am Coll Cardiol. 2009;54(8):686–94. Ted.
21. Herrmann HC, Rohatgi S, Wasserman HS, Block P, Gray W, Hamilton A, Zunamon A, Homma S, Di Tullio MR, Kraybill K, Merlino J, Martin R, Rodriguez L, Stewart WJ, Whitlow P, Wiegers SE, Silvestry FE, Foster E, Feldman T. Mitral valve hemodynamic effects of percuta-neous edge-to-edge repair with the MitraClip device for mitral regurgitation. Catheter Cardiovasc Interv. 2006;68:821–8.
22. Chandrashekhar Y, Westaby S, Narula J. Mitral stenosis. Lancet. 2009;74(9697):1271–83.
23. Nishimura RA, Otto CM, Bonow RO, Carabello BA, Erwin 3rd JP, Guyton RA, O'Gara PT, Ruiz CE, Skubas NJ, Sorajja P, Sundt 3rd TM, Thomas JD, American College of Cardiology/American Heart Association Task Force on Practice Guidelines. AHA/ACC guideline for the management of patients with valvular heart disease: executive summary: a report of the American College of Cardiology/American Heart Association Task Force on Practice Guidelines. J Am Coll Cardiol. 2014;63(22):2438–88.
24. Baumgartner H, Hung J, Bermejo J, Chambers JB, Evangelista A, Griffin BP, Iung B, Otto CM, Pellikka PA, Quiñones M, American Society of Echocardiography, European Association of Echocardiography. Echocardiographic assessment of valve stenosis: EAE/ASE recommen-dations for clinical practise. J Am Soc Echocardiogr. 2009;22(1):1–23.

25. Picano E, Pibarot P, Lancellotti P, Monin JL, Bonow RO. The emerging role of exercise testing and stress echocardiography in valvular heart disease. J Am Coll Cardiol. 2009;54(24): 2251–60.
26. Fino C, Iacovoni A, Ferrero P, Senni M, Merlo M, Cugola D, Ferrazzi P, Caputo M, Miceli A, Magne J. Restrictive mitral valve annuloplasty versus mitral valve replacement for functional ischemic mitral regurgitation: an exercise echocardiographic study. J Thorac Cardiovasc Surg. 2014;148(2):447–53.e2. doi:10.1016/j.jtcvs.2013.05.053. Epub 2013 Nov 4.
27. Chan KL, Chen SY, Chan V, Hay K, Mesana T, Lam BK. Functional significance of elevated mitral gradients after repair for degenerative mitral regurgitation. Circ Cardiovasc Imaging. 2013;6(6):1041–7.
28. Riegel AK, Bush R, Segal S, Fox JA, Eltzshing HK, Shernan SK. Evaluation of transmitral pressure gradients in the intraoperative echocardiographic diagnosis of mitral stenosis after mitral valve repair. PLoS One. 2011;6(11), e26559.
29. Armstrong WF, Ryan T. Feigenbaum's echocardiography. 7th ed. Philadelphia: Lippincott Williams and Wilkins; 2009.
30. Savage RM, Aronson S, Thomas JD, Shanewise JS, Shernan SK. Comprehensive textbook of intraoperative transesophageal echocardiography. Philadelphia: Lippincott Williams and Wilkins; 2004.

# Surgical Indications and Contraindications of the Edge-to-Edge

# 10

Alberto Pozzoli

## 10.1 Introduction

The edge-to-edge (EE) technique was introduced into the surgical armamentarium of mitral valve repair in the early 1990s and, from the beginning, it appeared to be an attractive approach because of its simplicity, reproducibility, and versatility [1, 2]. The surgical repair consists of suturing the free edge of the leaflets at the site of regurgitation, creating a valve with two orifices when the regurgitation originates from the middle scallops. The basic concept behind the EE approach is that the competence of the mitral valve can be effectively restored with a "functional" rather than an "anatomical" repair. As opposed to conventional techniques, mitral regurgitation is corrected by the obliteration of the regurgitant orifice at the leaflet level (echo-guided approach), regardless of the anatomical lesion. This concept implies that the same technique can be applied to different anatomical and functional conditions, to treat both organic and functional mitral regurgitation [2]. The largest experience of EE repair belongs to the San Raffaele University Hospital of Milan. The technique has been constantly refined over the years and has provided excellent results when correctly performed. Although the EE is a simple and versatile technique, several well-defined principles need to be rigorously respected in order to achieve efficacy and durability (Fig. 10.1).

A. Pozzoli
Department of Cardiac Surgery, IRCCS San Raffaele University Hospital,
Via Olgettina 60, Milan 20132, Italy
e-mail: albertopozzoli@gmail.com

© Springer International Publishing Switzerland 2015
O. Alfieri et al. (eds.), *Edge-to-Edge Mitral Repair: From a Surgical to a Percutaneous Approach*, DOI 10.1007/978-3-319-19893-4_10

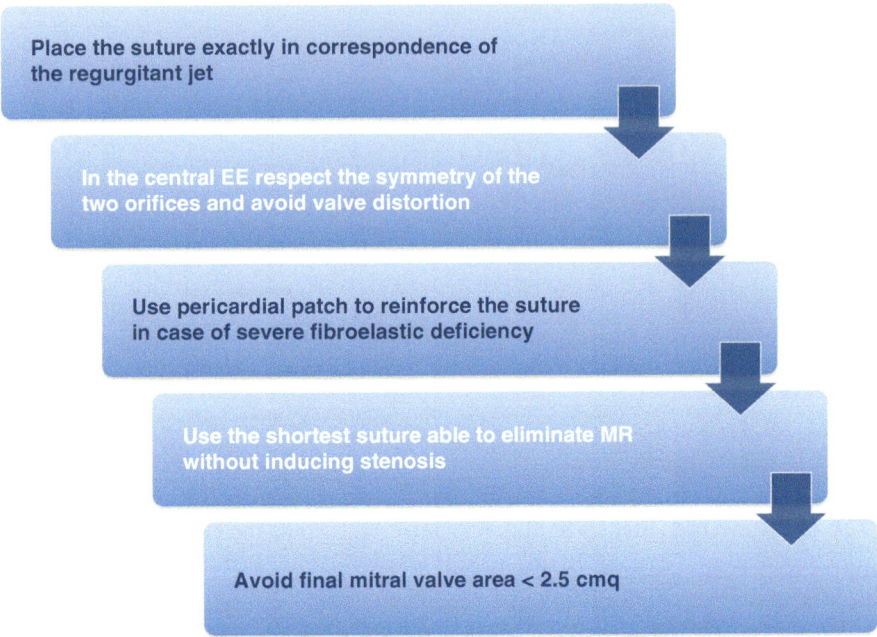

**Fig. 10.1** Technical key points in performing the EE repair

## 10.2  Current Indications of the Edge-to-Edge Mitral Valve Repair

Appropriate patient selection is crucial and transesophageal echocardiography (TEE) provides all the anatomical and functional features which are essentials for the EE repair. The current indications to the EE repair are essentially based on the surgical results obtained over the years in the different clinical settings (Fig. 10.2).

### 10.2.1 Bileaflet Prolapse of Facing Segments in Barlow's Disease

In patients with a global mixomatous degeneration of the mitral valve (Barlow's disease), all the components of the mitral apparatus are affected by a pathologic process which leads to generalized bileaflet prolapse and severe annular dilatation. In this context, the double-orifice EE repair has been applied as a standardized approach since 1993. Indeed, in most of the cases, the prolapse involves mainly the facing segments of the central portions of the anterior and posterior leaflets (A2 and P2) making it possible the surgical correction of MR by the EE technique. By suturing the middle scallop of the anterior and posterior leaflet (A2 to P2) followed by ring annuloplasty, the EE reduces the height of the leaflets in their middle portion,

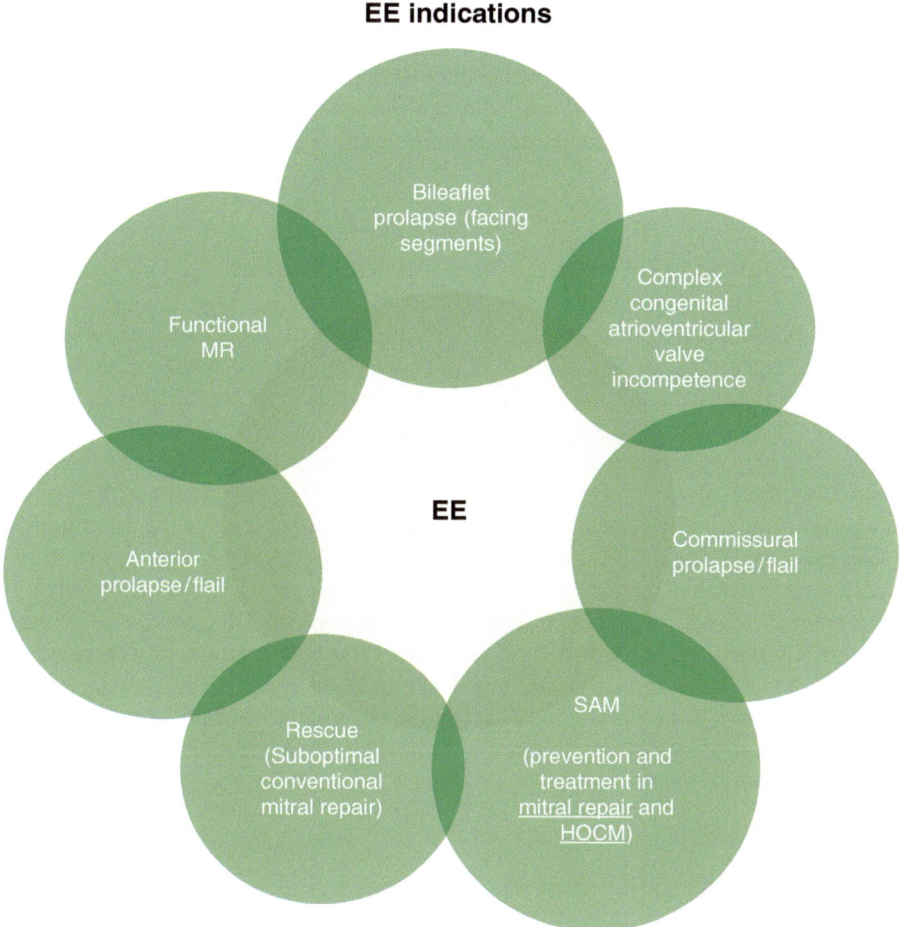

**Fig. 10.2**  Current indications of the EE technique

lowers the level of coaptation below the annulus, restores valve competence, and prevents postoperative systolic anterior movement (SAM).

A reduction of the global area of the mitral valve is the major drawback of this procedure. Such a reduction might be a disadvantage when the technique is applied on valves without annular dilatation, while it is usually not a problem in the setting of Barlow's disease. Leaflet redundancy, especially of the posterior leaflet, predisposes to postoperative left ventricular outflow obstruction due to systolic anterior movement (SAM) of the anterior leaflet when conventional techniques of repair are applied in Barlow's disease. Sliding plasty of the posterior leaflet is necessary to reduce this risk. The double-orifice technique abolishes the risk of SAM by fixing the free edge of the anterior leaflet in the area usually responsible for this phenomenon. The technique provides a safe and predictable result by a simple and standardized procedure.

The clinical and echocardiographic long-term results of the EE correction in this subset, proved that the double-orifice technique in combination with ring annuloplasty provides excellent late outcomes both in terms of freedom from reoperation and from recurrent MR [3].

## 10.2.2 Segmental Prolapse of the Anterior Leaflet

Unlike posterior leaflet prolapse which can be easily repaired with excellent outcomes, prolapse of the anterior leaflet has been traditionally associated to decreased repair rate and higher late failure, even in experienced centers [4, 5]. This mechanism of MR can be typically found in patients with anterior leaflet chordal elongation or rupture in the setting of degenerative mitral valve disorder (myxomatous disease or fibroelastic deficiency) or postendocarditis mitral regurgitation. If only one scallop (usually A2) is prolapsing, the EE repair is very effective in restoring mitral valve competence in a rapid, standardized, and easily reproducible manner [6]. However, in presence of extended prolapse of the anterior leaflet involving more than one scallop, the EE approach might not be sufficient to obtain a perfectly competent valve, because a long suture would be required with a high risk of mitral stenosis. In those circumstances, other techniques should be preferred, or artificial chordae should be added to the EE repair to eliminate incompetence, without excessively reducing the valve area [5, 7, 8].

## 10.2.3 Commissural Prolapse

Several technically demanding methods of repair were described for the treatment of commissural prolapse. The absence of a unique and standardized approach in this context demonstrates the challenging feature of "commissural mitral regurgitation." In addition, the frailty of the valve tissue at this level further increases the complexity of the reconstruction. Complete suturing of the entire commissural area of prolapse (paracommissural EE) followed by annuloplasty, effectively eliminates prolapse, regardless of the fact that the anterior, posterior, or both leaflets are involved [9, 10]. From a technical point of view, the paracommissural EE repair (also called commissural closure) consists of the complete suturing of the entire commissural area of prolapse. The long-term results of this procedure in our experience are extremely satisfactory in patients with degenerative or postendocarditis prolapse or flail of the commissural mitral region [11]. Those results, up to 15 years after the operation, validated the EE technique as a simple and reproducible method to repair isolated commissural prolapse or flail.

### 10.2.4 Secondary Mitral Regurgitation

An undersized annuloplasty with a complete rigid ring is the standard operation in severe symptomatic secondary MR. However, mitral insufficiency can recur in a significant number of cases and the durability of such a procedure seems to be particularly unreliable in patients with mild-to-moderate annular dilatation, severe tethering, and complex jets. Surely, if substantial apical tenting is present (coaptation depth >1 cm), ring annuloplasty alone may not be sufficient. In these patients with a more advanced degree of leaflet tethering, the EE technique may play an important role in addiction to annuloplasty to enhance the likelihood of a durable repair [12]. The rationale for using the EE technique in functional MR is that, with this approach, the site of the regurgitant jet is specifically addressed and early valve closure is ensured. Moreover, by anchoring the leaflets together, the EE might counteract the progression of the LV remodeling with a kind of "rein" effect. The preoperative echocardiographic study has literally to be used as a guide to identify the site of the approximating stitch which is chosen according to the echocardiographic location of the major regurgitant jet. When more than one regurgitant jet is present, the EE is applied on the largest one, relying on the undersized ring for the resolution of the others. The length of the suture is always kept very short to minimize the risk of postoperative mitral valve stenosis. A complete rigid or semirigid prosthetic ring is invariably implanted. In the setting of functional mitral regurgitation it is usually one or two sizes smaller than the anterior leaflet surface.

### 10.2.5 EE to Prevent Systolic Anterior Motion (SAM) After Mitral Repair and in Patients with Hypertrophic Obstructive Cardiomyopathy (HOCM)

The use of the EE technique can be very effective in treating postoperative systolic anterior motion (SAM) in patients undergoing mitral valve repair [13]. The technique can be safely used for this purpose, avoiding more complicated and time consuming alternatives such as annuloplasty ring removal, use of a larger ring or neochordae implantation. The same approach can be adopted to prevent this complication in patients who have high risk of post-repair SAM and left ventricular outflow tract obstruction [14].

The double-orifice technique is also indicated to prevent the occurrence of left ventricular outflow obstruction in patients with hypertrophic obstructive cardiomyopathy (HOCM) and residual SAM after septal myectomy [15].

### 10.2.6 EE as "Rescue" Technique

Another useful indication of the EE technique is represented by its use to "rescue" patients with significant residual MR after conventional mitral repair ("rescue EE").

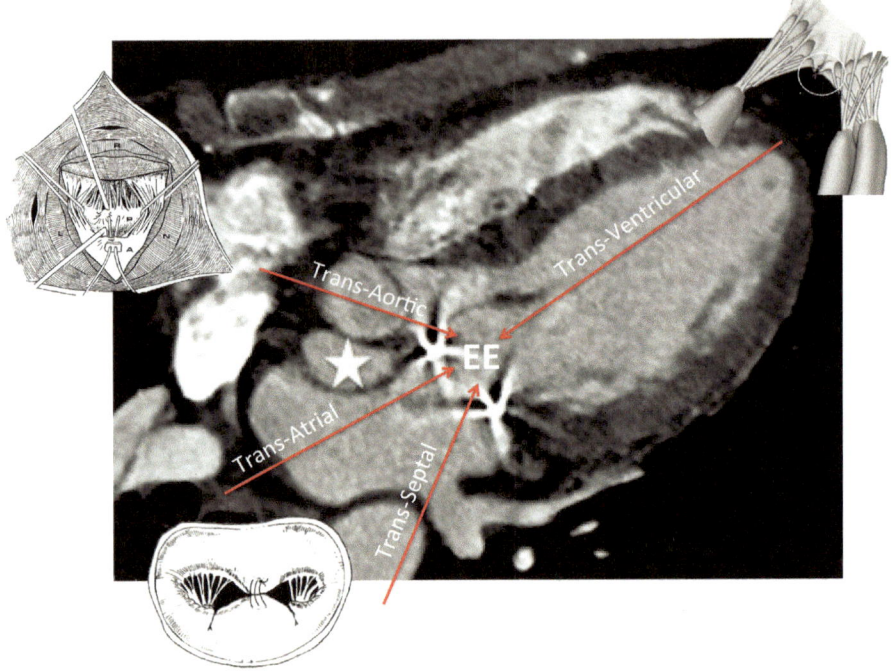

**Fig. 10.3** Possible surgical accesses to perform the EE repair

The absence of residual MR immediately after the procedure is extremely important for the long-term durability of the repair. The most frequent causes of immediate MV repair failure are left ventricular outflow tract obstruction due to SAM, incomplete repair (residual prolapse, inadequate annuloplasty, clefts), and suture dehiscence. The rescue EE requires only few more minutes of aortic cross-clamp time since it can be performed without taking down the initial repair. The residual regurgitant jet is addressed exactly where it is identified by saline solution test or postoperative TEE. The Columbia Presbyterian Hospital reported the first series of patients treated with a "rescue EE" [16]. In our experience mitral valves rescued by an EE suture after a suboptimal conventional repair maintained their competence at long-term [17].

### 10.2.7 Transaortic EE Repair of MR

Another interesting application of the EE is in the context of less than severe MR in high risk patients undergoing aortic valve surgery. In this context, the addition of mitral valve surgery to aortic valve replacement (AVR) significantly increases the operative risk. In selected patients, an EE repair of the mitral valve can be performed through the aortic valve, before the AVR (Fig. 10.3). It is a simple way to improve MR without adding significant time or complexity to the procedure [18]. Of course an annuloplasty ring cannot be implanted limiting the durability of the repair. Therefore this solution should be considered as a "compromise" to be accepted only in very high risk/old patients.

## 10.2.8  Special Settings

The EE repair may also be used in the following very selected situations:

- Children with complex congenital heart disease associated with atrioventricular valve incompetence [19];
- Patients in whom mitral valve exposure is extremely difficult (deep chest, small left atrium, severe LV hypertrophy, dilated aortic root);
- During LV reconstruction operations since the EE repair can be carried out through the left ventriculotomy in case of concomitant mitral regurgitation [20, 21] (Fig. 10.3);
- In patients with severe left ventricular dysfunction or need for concomitant multiple procedures in whom the EE is particularly convenient due to the short aortic cross-clamp time required.

## 10.2.9  Minimally Invasive Mitral Valve Repair

Finally, this technique is certainly very appealing, due to its technical simplicity, when a minimally invasive approach is adopted to treat MR [22, 23].

## 10.3   Contraindications

Despite this great versatility, clinical and echocardiographic results progressively demonstrated that there are specific subgroups of patients in whom the EE technique leads to suboptimal results. It should be avoided in presence of heavily calcified annulus and whenever annular dilatation cannot be corrected by a concomitant annuloplasty for whatever reason. Indeed, the absence of annuloplasty is likely associated with increased stresses on the suture and on the valve apparatus, leading to accelerated failure of the repair [24, 25]. Unsatisfactory outcomes have been reported also in patients with rheumatic mitral regurgitation [2].

Because of the risk of inducing stenosis, the EE technique should not be used in patients with small mitral valve area. In addition, its application is not indicated in case of bileaflet prolapse if the mitral lesions involve not facing segments. In the above mentioned conditions the EE repair does not represent the technique of choice (Fig. 10.4).

## EE Contraindications

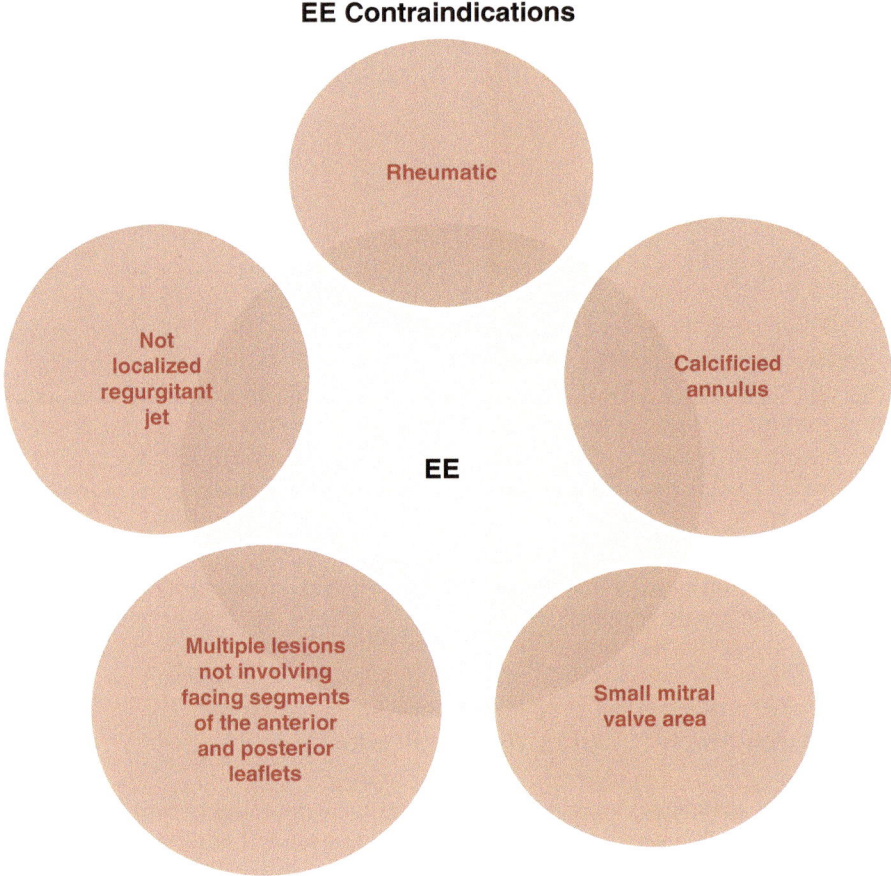

**Fig. 10.4** Current contraindications of the EE technique

### Conclusion

Twenty years after its introduction, the edge-to-edge technique has been tested and performed worldwide by several institutions and it remains an effective and versatile method to treat mitral regurgitation due to different causes and mechanisms. Simplicity, reliability and reproducibility are the main advantages of this method. Very long-term durability has recently been definitely demonstrated. The current indications and contraindications of the edge-to-edge repair, substantiated by the surgical results, have been outlined in this chapter. If the well-established technical aspects of the procedure are respected and the precise patient selection criteria are observed, results with this type of repair are similar or even superior to those obtained with other reconstructive techniques.

# References

1. Fucci C, Sandrelli L, Pardini A, et al. Improved results with mitral valve repair using new surgical techniques. Eur J Cardiothorac Surg. 1995;9:621–6.
2. Alfieri O, Maisano F, De Bonis M, et al. The double-orifice technique in mitral valve repair: a simple solution for complex problems. J Thorac Cardiovasc Surg. 2001;122:674–81.
3. De Bonis M, Lapenna E, Lorusso R, Buzzatti N, Gelsomino S, Taramasso M, Vizzardi E, Alfieri O. Very long-term results (up to 17 years) with the double-orifice mitral valve repair combined with ring annuloplasty for degenerative mitral regurgitation. J Thorac Cardiovasc Surg. 2012;144(5):1019–24.
4. Seeburger J, Borger MA, Doll N, Walther T, Passage J, Falk V, et al. Comparison of outcomes of minimally invasive mitral valve surgery for posterior, anterior and bileaflet prolapse. Eur J Cardiothorac Surg. 2009;36:532–8.
5. David TE, Armstrong S, Ivanov J. Chordal replacement with polytetrafluoroethylene sutures for mitral valve repair: a 25-year experience. J Thorac Cardiovasc Surg. 2013;145:1563–9.
6. Alfieri O, Maisano F. An effective technique to correct anterior mitral leaflet prolapse. J Card Surg. 1999;14:468–70.
7. De Bonis M, Lorusso R, Lapenna E, Kassem S, De Cicco G, Torracca L, Maisano F, La Canna G, Alfieri O. Similar long-term results of mitral valve repair for anterior compared with posterior leaflet prolapse. J Thorac Cardiovasc Surg. 2006;131(2):364–70. Epub 2006 Jan 18.
8. De Bonis M, Lapenna E, Taramasso M, La Canna G, Buzzatti N, Pappalardo F, Alfieri O. Very long-term durability of the edge-to-edge repair for isolated anterior mitral leaflet prolapse: up to 21 years of clinical and echocardiographic results. J Thorac Cardiovasc Surg. 2014;27.
9. Gillinov AM, Shortt KG, Cosgrove 3rd DM. Commissural closure for repair of mitral commissural prolapse. Ann Thorac Surg. 2005;80:1135–6.
10. Lapenna E, De Bonis M, Sorrentino F, La Canna G, Grimaldi A, Torracca L, et al. Commissural closure for the treatment of commissural mitral valve prolapse or flail. J Heart Valve Dis. 2008;17:261–6.
11. De Bonis M, Lapenna E, Taramasso M, Pozzoli A, La Canna G, Calabrese MC, Alfieri O. Is commissural closure associated with mitral annuloplasty a durable technique for the treatment of mitral regurgitation? A long-term ($\leq$15 years) clinical and echocardiographic study. J Thorac Cardiovasc Surg. 2014;147(6):1900–6.
12. De Bonis M, Lapenna E, La Canna G, et al. Mitral valve repair for functional mitral regurgitation in end-stage dilated cardiomyopathy: role of the "edge-to-edge" technique. Circulation. 2005;112:402–8.
13. Myers PO, Khalpey Z, Maloney AM, et al. Edge-to-edge repair for prevention and treatment of mitral valve systolic anterior motion. J Thorac Cardiovasc Surg. 2013;146(4):836–40.
14. Mascagni R, Al Attar N, Lamarra M, et al. Edge-to-edge technique to treat post-mitral valve repair systolic anterior motion and left ventricular outflow tract obstruction. Ann Thorac Surg. 2005;79:471–3.
15. Wan CK, Dearani JA, Sundt 3rd TM, et al. What is the best surgical treatment for obstructive hypertrophic cardiomyopathy and degenerative mitral regurgitation? Ann Thorac Surg. 2009;88:727–31.
16. Kherani AR, Cheema FH, Casher J, et al. Edge-to-edge mitral valve repair: the Columbia Presbyterian experience. Ann Thorac Surg. 2004;78:73–6.
17. De Bonis M, Lapenna E, Buzzatti N, et al. Can the edge-to-edge technique provide durable results when used to rescue patients with suboptimal conventional mitral repair? Eur J Cardiothorac Surg. 2013;43:173–9.
18. Mihos CG, Santana O, Brenes JC, Lamelas J. Outcomes of transaortic edge-to-edge repair of the mitral valve in patients undergoing minimally invasive aortic valve replacement. J Thorac Cardiovasc Surg. 2013;145(5):1412–3.

19. Ando M, Takahashi Y. Edge-to-edge repair of common atrioventricular or tricuspid valve in patients with functionally single ventricle. Ann Thorac Surg. 2007;84:1571–6.
20. McCarthy PM, Starling RC, Wong J, et al. Early results with partial left ventriculectomy. J Thorac Cardiovasc Surg. 1997;114:755–63.
21. McCarthy JF, McCarthy PM, Starling RC, Smedira NG, Scalia GM, Wong J, Kasirajan V, Goormastic M, Young JB. Partial left ventriculectomy and mitral valve repair for end-stage congestive heart failure. Eur J Cardiothoracic Surg. 1998;13:337–43.
22. Lapenna E, Torracca L, De Bonis M, et al. Minimally invasive mitral valve repair in the context of Barlow's disease. Ann Thorac Surg. 2005;79:1496–9.
23. Glower DD, Desai B, Mackensen GB. Early results of edge-to-edge Alfieri mitral repair via right mini-thoracotomy in 68 consecutive patients. Innovations (Phila). 2009;4:256–60.
24. Maisano F, Caldarola A, Blasio A, et al. Midterm results of edge-to-edge mitral valve repair without annuloplasty. J Thorac Cardiovasc Surg. 2003;126:1987–97.
25. De Bonis M, Lapenna E, Maisano F, Barili F, La Canna G, Buzzatti N, Pappalardo F, Calabrese M, Nisi T, Alfieri O. Long-term results (≤18 years) of the edge-to-edge mitral valve repair without annuloplasty in degenerative mitral regurgitation: implications for the percutaneous approach. Circulation. 2014;130(11 Suppl 1):S19–24.

# The Case of Surgical Edge-to-Edge Repair Without Annuloplasty: Now We Know

11

Elisabetta Lapenna, Davide Schiavi, Gabriele Del Castillo, and Michele De Bonis

In degenerative mitral regurgitation (MR), annuloplasty is commonly recommended to complete mitral valve (MV) repair. Particularly when a prosthetic ring is used, this procedure stabilizes the reconstruction over time by increasing leaflet coaptation and preventing re-dilatation of the mitral annulus [1–4]. Several studies have reported that the absence of annuloplasty is one of the most important risk factor for late failure of the repair in degenerative MR [1–4]. The important role of the annuloplasty procedure becomes even more crucial when the edge-to-edge (EE) technique is used. Indeed, in the degenerative setting, the EE technique provides excellent freedom from reoperation and recurrence of MR at long-term when combined with a concomitant annuloplasty [5–7]. However, less satisfactory results have been documented whenever the annuloplasty is missed for whatever reason [8–12].

## 11.1  Computational Models Data

By using computational models, Votta and coworkers were able to simulate and assess the stress pattern occurring on the MV structures both in systole and in diastole after an EE repair [13]. This model showed that, while in the native mitral valve diastolic stresses are negligible, after the EE repair diastolic peak stresses are comparable to those calculated in systole and depend on the size of the annulus. Therefore, after an EE technique, the valve components are exposed to a systolic

E. Lapenna • D. Schiavi • G. Del Castillo
Department of Cardiac Surgery, IRCCS San Raffaele University Hospital, Milan, Italy

M. De Bonis, MD (✉)
Department of Cardiac Surgery, IRCCS San Raffaele University Hospital, Milan, Italy

Department of Cardiac Surgery, San Raffaele Scientific Institute,
Via Olgettina 60, 20132 Milan, Italy
e-mail: debonis.michele@hsr.it

© Springer International Publishing Switzerland 2015
O. Alfieri et al. (eds.), *Edge-to-Edge Mitral Repair: From a Surgical to a Percutaneous Approach*, DOI 10.1007/978-3-319-19893-4_11

stress that is twice the one occurring in a native mitral valve. Furthermore, it was found that a 20 % dilation of the annulus intensifies the stresses both in the annular region and close to the EE suture. This last finding clearly indicates that the lack of annuloplasty is associated with increased stresses on the suture and on the leaflets, possibly leading to accelerated failure of the EE reconstruction. Therefore, according to this model, a concomitant annuloplasty represents a key factor for the long-term durability of the EE repair.

## 11.2    Clinical Data

In the clinical setting, initially, a retrospective analysis was conducted in 2001 in a group of 260 patients submitted to the double-orifice repair [8]. Patients who had a ringless EE reconstruction showed a higher failure rate compared to patients who received a concomitant annuloplasty. The freedom from reoperation at 5 years was 70 % ± 15 % vs 92 % ± 3.4 %, respectively ($P = 0.02$) [8].

A subsequent analysis carried out on 81 patients submitted to EE mitral repair without associated annuloplasty [9], confirmed those preliminary findings but, in addition, demonstrated that midterm results (≤5 years) were particularly poor in patients with calcified annulus and in those who showed more than mild residual MR at hospital discharge [9]. However, the study population was very heterogeneous, including primarily patients with degenerative MR but also cases of functional, rheumatic, and post-endocarditis mitral insufficiency. In most of those cases a contraindication for annuloplasty was present, more often annular calcification, and the EE technique was used to treat complex lesions such as anterior and bileaflet prolapse, restrictive leaflet motion, and leaflet erosions due to endocarditis. When patients with a severely calcified annulus, rheumatic lesions, or rescue EE were excluded, results were rather encouraging, suggesting that a ringless EE might offer adequate mid-term results, provided that annular function is preserved and the indication for the EE technique is correct.

This finding was certainly interesting and represented the background for a further clinical and echocardiographic analysis of a selected subgroup of 29 patients, with either degenerative or functional MR, in whom annuloplasty was intentionally not added to isolated central EE repair because of limited annular dilatation/distortion [10]. Patients with severe annular calcification were excluded from the study as well as those with rheumatic valve disease, obstructive cardiomyopathy, or endocarditis, in whom repair results would likely be influenced by the cause of the MR itself. In this selected group of patients with a relatively preserved anatomy and function of the mitral annulus, the 5-year freedom from reoperation or recurrence of MR ≥ 3+ was 90 ± 5 %, although at a median follow-up of 6.3 years, about one-third of patients showed a tendency toward MR progression. According to the findings of this study, the surgical EE mitral repair, intentionally performed without annuloplasty, appeared to have acceptable mid-term results. And what about the long-term outcomes? Only recently the long-term results of the ringless EE repair have become available [11]. These data are rather unique because the EE technique was

**Fig. 11.1** Overall survival (With permission for reprint from *Curr Opin Cardiol.* 2015 Jan 8 [Epub ahead of print])

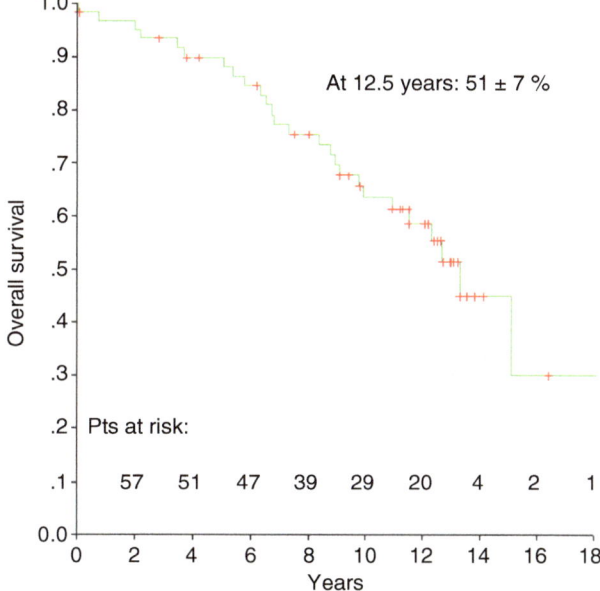

introduced in the early 1990s [14] and there are no other series available including patients with surgical ringless EE repair followed for a median time of 9 years (up to 18 years). The population of this last study includes 61 patients with degenerative MR due to bileaflet prolapse (46 % of the cases), anterior leaflet prolapse (18 %), and prolapse of the posterior leaflet (36 %). The main reason for annuloplasty omission was the presence of either important annular calcification or limited annular dilatation/deformation. In case of significantly/severely calcified annulus, which was present in 36 patients (59 %), the rationale for adopting the EE technique was to correct leaflet lesions with no annular manipulation. In the remaining 25 patients (41 %), the EE was intentionally performed without a concomitant annuloplasty because the annulus was judged by the surgeon not to be significantly dilated. By avoiding annuloplasty in those cases, also the risk of inducing postoperative mitral stenosis was minimized.

Hospital mortality was 1.6 %. Follow-up was complete. In the two subgroups mentioned above, mean clinical and echocardiographic follow-up time was 9.2±4.2 years (median 9.7) and 7.4±3.4 years (median 8, longest 18 years), respectively. At 12 years, overall survival was 51±7 % (Fig. 11.1), freedom from cardiac death 87±4.5 % (Fig. 11.2), and freedom from reoperation due to repair failure was 57.8±7.21 % (Fig. 11.3). When freedom from reoperation was assessed according to the presence of annular calcification, at mid-term (up to 4 years after surgery) patients without calcification had less events compared to those with annular calcification (85±7.6 % vs. 76±7.2 %). However, beyond that time frame, no statistically significant differences were observed (at 9 years 58.6±11.4 % vs. 57.8±9.14 %, $P=0.7$) (Fig. 11.4).

**Fig. 11.2** Freedom from cardiac death (With permission for reprint from [11])

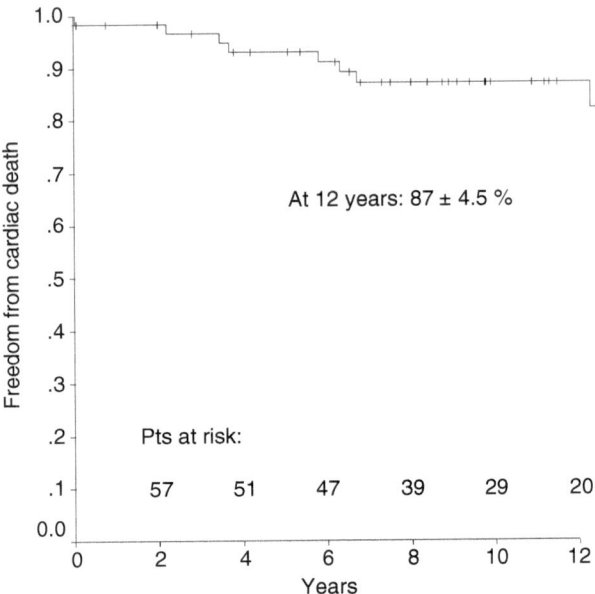

**Fig. 11.3** Freedom from reoperation (With permission for reprint from [11])

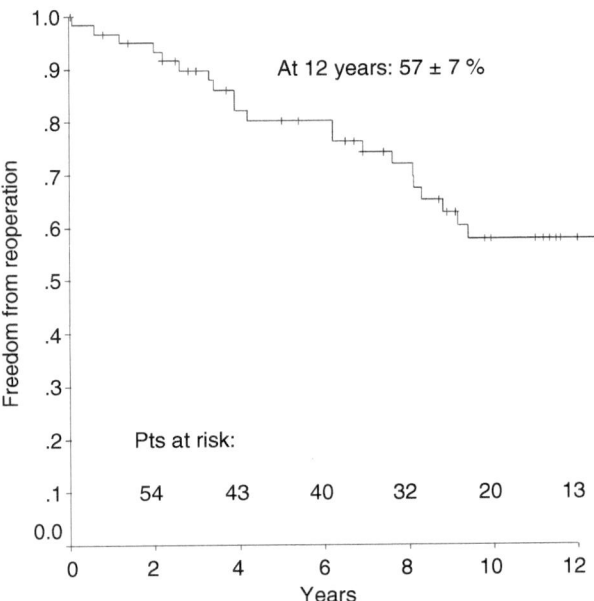

At the last echocardiographic assessment 55 % of the hospital survivors had MR≥3+. Freedom from MR≥3+ at 12 years was 43±7.6 % (Fig. 11.5). Interestingly, as for the reoperation rate, patients without annular calcifications showed at mid-term (≤4 years) a higher freedom from recurrent MR 3+ or 4+ (81±8.4 %) compared with those in whom annuloplasty was omitted for the presence of important

**Fig. 11.4** Freedom from reoperation in patients with and without annular calcification (With permission for reprint from *Curr Opin Cardiol.* 2015 Jan 8)

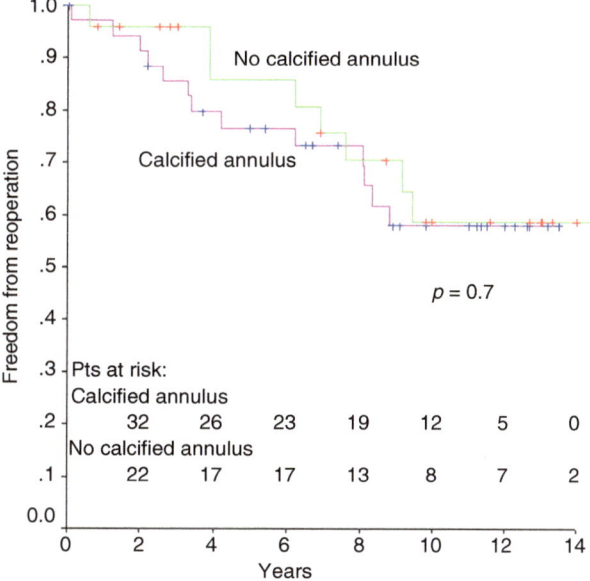

**Fig. 11.5** Freedom from recurrence of MR of grade 3 to 4+ (With permission for reprint from [11])

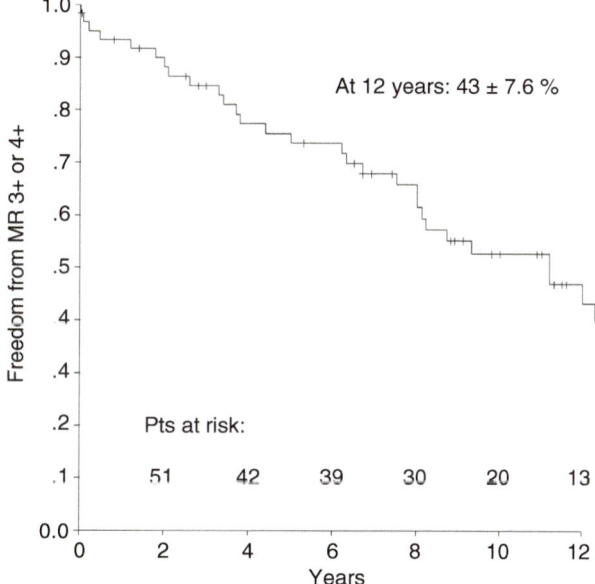

calcification ($73 \pm 7.5$ %). With increased follow-up length, however, no statistically significant differences could be demonstrated between the two groups (at 9 years $54 \pm 11.4$ % vs. $52 \pm 8.8$ %, $P = 0.1$; Fig. 11.6). In addition, this study showed that an initial suboptimal result (residual MR > 1+/4+ at hospital discharge) was a significant risk factor for recurrent MR 3+ or 4+ at follow-up. When the initial result was

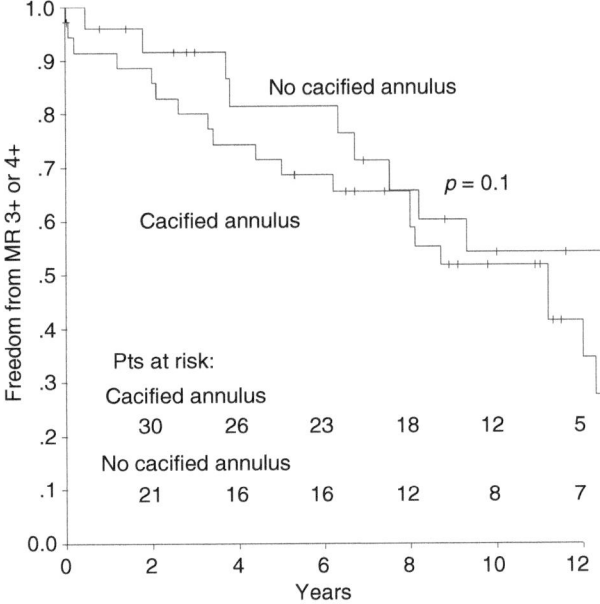

**Fig. 11.6** Freedom from recurrence of MR of grade 3 to 4+ in patients with and without annular calcification (With permission for reprint from [11])

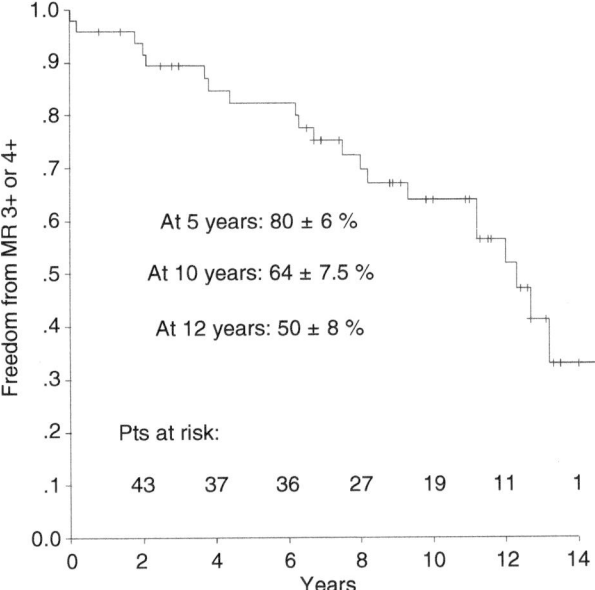

**Fig. 11.7** Freedom from reoperation and recurrence of MR of grade 3 to 4+ in patients with initial optimal result (residual MR 0 or 1+/4+) at hospital discharge (With permission for reprint from *Curr Opin Cardiol.* 2015 Jan 8)

optimal (MR 0 or 1+), freedom from MR ≥3+/4+ was better compared to the entire study population but still rather disappointing being 50±8 % at 12 years (Fig. 11.7). Finally, freedom from recurrent MR ≥3+ was explored also for the best possible subgroup of patients, which means for the only 24 patients with intentionally avoided annuloplasty (no annular calcification) and with no or mild residual MR at hospital discharge. In those patients, freedom from this event was $62.8 \pm 11.2$ % at 9 years.

## 11.3   Comment

There are several lessons which have been learned from the experience accumulated so far with the ringless EE mitral valve repair:

1. In degenerative MR, the overall long-term results of the surgical EE technique without annuloplasty are not satisfactory. A concomitant annuloplasty, therefore, represents a key factor for the long-term durability of the EE repair;
2. The EE repair performed without a concomitant annuloplasty is not effective in the challenging setting of extensively calcified annulus and MR due to myxomatous disease. Under those circumstances, alternative approaches, including mitral repair with annular decalcification followed by ring annuloplasty or mitral valve replacement should be preferred [15–19];
3. In patients with degenerative MR without annular calcification, in whom prosthetic annuloplasty is intentionally avoided because of only mild annular dilatation/deformation, the ringless EE repair provides acceptable results at mid-term but is associated with a high failure rate at long-term. This is possibly due to the progression of the degenerative disease leading to further annular enlargement.

Those findings may be of some interest in the current "Mitraclip era," considering the fact that, so far, around 20,000 patients have been treated worldwide with a percutaneous trans-catheter EE approach without a concomitant annuloplasty [12, 20, 21]. They emphasize the importance of an appropriate selection of the MitraClip candidates in order to minimize residual MR after the procedure. In addition they underline the need for a reliable trans-catheter annuloplasty [22] to improve the long-term outcomes of the currently available percutaneous EE procedure.

## References

1. Gillinov AM, Tantiwongkosri K, Blackstone EH, et al. Is prosthetic annuloplasty necessary for durable mitral valve repair? Ann Thorac Surg. 2009;88:76–82.
2. Gillinov AM, Cosgrove DM, Blackstone EH, et al. Durability of mitral valve repair for degenerative disease. J Thorac Cardiovasc Surg. 1998;116:734–43.
3. Flameng W, Herijgers P, Bogaerts K. Recurrence of mitral regurgitation after mitral valve repair in degenerative valve disease. Circulation. 2003;107:1609–13.
4. David TE, Armstrong S, McCrindle BW, Manlhiot C. Late outcomes of mitral valve repair for mitral regurgitation due to degenerative disease. Circulation. 2013;127:1485–92.
5. De Bonis M, Lapenna E, Taramasso M, et al. Very long-term durability of the edge-to-edge repair for isolated anterior mitral leaflet prolapse: up to 21 years of clinical and echocardiographic results. J Thorac Cardiovasc Surg. 2014;148(5):2027–32.

6. De Bonis M, Lapenna E, Taramasso M, et al. Is commissural closure associated with mitral annuloplasty a durable technique for the treatment of mitral regurgitation? A long-term (≤15 years) clinical and echocardiographic study. J Thorac Cardiovasc Surg. 2014;147:1900–6.

7. De Bonis M, Lapenna E, Lorusso R, et al. Very long-term results (up to 17 years) with the double-orifice mitral valve repair combined with ring annuloplasty for degenerative mitral regurgitation. J Thorac Cardiovasc Surg. 2012;144:1019–24.

8. Alfieri O, Maisano F, De Bonis M, et al. The double-orifice technique in mitral valve repair: a simple solution for complex problems. J Thorac Cardiovasc Surg. 2001;122:674–81.

9. Maisano F, Caldarola A, Blasio A, et al. Midterm results of edge-to-edge mitral valve repair without annuloplasty. J Thorac Cardiovasc Surg. 2003;126:1987–97.

10. Maisano F, Viganò G, Blasio A, et al. Surgical isolated edge-to-edge mitral valve repair without annuloplasty: clinical proof of the principle for an endovascular approach. EuroIntervention. 2006;2:181–6.

11. De Bonis M, Lapenna E, Maisano F, et al. Long-term results (≤18 years) of the edge-to-edge mitral valve repair without annuloplasty in degenerative mitral regurgitation: implications for the percutaneous approach. Circulation. 2014;130(11 Suppl 1):S19–24.

12. De Bonis M, Lapenna E, Pozzoli A, et al. Edge-to-edge surgical mitral valve repair in the era of MitraClip: what if the annuloplasty ring is missed? Curr Opin Cardiol. 2015 Jan 8. [Epub ahead of print].

13. Votta E, Maisano F, Soncini M, et al. 3-D computational analysis of the stress distribution on the leaflets after edge-to-edge repair of mitral regurgitation. J Heart Valve Dis. 2002;11:810–22.

14. Fucci C, Sandrelli L, Pardini A, et al. Improved results with mitral valve repair using new surgical techniques. Eur J Cardiothorac Surg. 1995;9:621–6.

15. Feindel CM, Tufail Z, David TE, Ivanov J, Armstrong S. Mitral valve surgery in patients with extensive calcification of the mitral annulus. J Thorac Cardiovasc Surg. 2003;126:777–82.

16. Carpentier AF, Pellerin M, Fuzellier JF, Relland JY. Extensive calcification of the mitral valve annulus: pathology and surgical management. J Thorac Cardiovasc Surg. 1996;111:718–29.

17. David TE, Feindel CM, Armstrong S, Sun Z. Reconstruction of the mitral anulus. A ten-year experience. J Thorac Cardiovasc Surg. 1995;110:1323–32.

18. Fasol R, Mahdjoobian K, Joubert-Hubner E. Mitral repair in patients with severely calcified annulus: feasibility, surgery and results. J Heart Valve Dis. 2002;11:153–9.

19. Ng CK, Punzengruber C, Pachinger O, et al. Valve repair in mitral regurgitation complicated by severe annulus calcification. Ann Thorac Surg. 2000;70:53–8.

20. Maisano F, Franzen O, Baldus S, et al. Percutaneous mitral valve interventions in the real world: early and 1-year results from the ACCESS-EU, a prospective, multicenter, nonrandomized post-approval study of the MitraClip therapy in Europe. J Am Coll Cardiol. 2013; 62:1052–61.

21. Mauri L, Foster E, Glower DD, et al. EVEREST II Investigators. 4-year results of a randomized controlled trial of percutaneous repair versus surgery for mitral regurgitation. J Am Coll Cardiol. 2013;62(4):317–28.

22. Taramasso M, Maisano F. Transcatheter mitral valve repair – transcatheter mitral valve annuloplasty. EuroIntervention. 2014;10 Suppl U:U129–35.

# Evolution of the Edge-to-Edge Repair: From a Surgical to a Percutaneous Approach

# 12

Stefano Benussi, Alberto Pozzoli, Maurizio Taramasso, and Paolo Denti

The edge-to-edge (EE) is a surgical technique developed by Alfieri [1–3] in the early 1990s to treat mitral regurgitation (MR). The technique is quite easily performed and it is used to treat both organic and functional MR. The surgical procedure consists of the suture of the free edge of the leaflets at the site of regurgitation (Fig. 12.1). As opposed to conventional techniques, the EE repair is not directly addressing the anatomical lesion because MR is corrected by obliteration of the regurgitant orifice at the leaflet level. Actually the strategy leads to a new different functional anatomy as a trade-off for the old dysfunctional valve. This innovative concept implies the versatility of the technique, which can be applied to different anatomical and functional conditions. Many years ago, we predicted that the EE repair, due to its simplicity, could open the perspective of percutaneous correction of MR [3]. The prediction became reality, and nowadays the EE concept is the basis of the currently most widespread and successful catheter-based technologies of correcting MR, the MitraClip (Abbott Vascular, Inc., Menlo Park, California). From a historical perspective, this is perhaps the greatest merit of the edge-to-edge technique.

S. Benussi (✉) • M. Taramasso
Cardiac Surgery, University Hospital Zurich, Rämistrasse 100, Zurich 8091, Switzerland
e-mail: stefano.benussi@usz.ch; m.taramasso@gmail.com

A. Pozzoli • P. Denti
Department of Cardiac Surgery, IRCCS San Raffaele University Hospital,
Via Olgettina 60, Milan 20132, Italy
e-mail: albertopozzoli@gmail.com; denti.paolo@hsr.it

© Springer International Publishing Switzerland 2015
O. Alfieri et al. (eds.), *Edge-to-Edge Mitral Repair: From a Surgical to a Percutaneous Approach*, DOI 10.1007/978-3-319-19893-4_12

129

**Fig. 12.1** Surgical
application of the edge-to-
edge technique

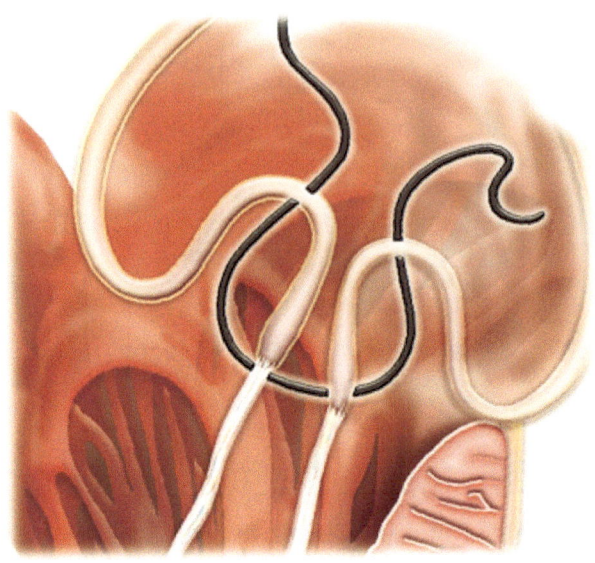

## 12.1    Surgical Edge-to-Edge Without the Addition of Annuloplasty

Annuloplasty is routinely performed in surgical mitral repair as it has been clearly demonstrated to improve early and long-term results [4]. The same applies to patients undergoing open surgical repair with the EE technique: in the overall population, the absence of annuloplasty is associated with shorter durability of the repair [1]. In a focused study, Alfieri et al. [1] reported shorter durability in patients treated with his repair, without annuloplasty. However, these patients usually had conditions preventing ring implantation that could directly influence durability, such as annular calcification, endocarditic or rheumatic disease, a previously failed attempt of repair, or they were operated in the setting of minimally invasive and robotic interventions. The outcomes of 81 patients treated by EE technique without annuloplasty showed an overall survival of $85 \pm 7$ % and a freedom from reoperation at 4 years of $89 \pm 3.9$ %. Annular calcification was associated with a higher reoperation rate ($77 \pm 22$ % vs. $95 \pm 4.6$ % in the calcified vs. noncalcified annulus, $p = 0.03$). Late failure was predicted by early residual MR assessed either by saline testing or intraoperative trans-esophageal echocardiography (TEE) [5]. In the absence of annular calcification or complex anatomy (rheumatic disease, endocarditis, rescue repair), midterm durability of the isolated EE was acceptable, as confirmed by the 5-year outcomes of selected subgroup of patients with ideal anatomy treated without annuloplasty [6]. These findings were at that time the clinical proof of concept for the isolated percutaneous treatment. At long-term the results change: as recently reported by De Bonis et al., at 12 years the freedom from reoperation was $57.8 \pm 7.21$ % and freedom from recurrence of MR $\geq$3+ was $43 \pm 7.6$ %. Importantly, in patients with residual MR $\leq$1+ immediately after surgery, freedom from MR $\geq$3+ at 5 and 10 years was $80 \pm 6$ % and $64 \pm 7.58$ %, respectively. Early optimal competence (residual MR $\leq$1+) was associated with higher freedom from recurrent severe regurgitation. These results outlined that the long-term results of the surgical EE technique without annuloplasty are not satisfactory in degenerative MR. Eventually, the future addition of a percutaneous annuloplasty would improve clinical results and further expand the indications for trans-catheter mitral valve EE.

## 12.2   The Transition from a Surgical Procedure to the Trans-catheter Approach

In 1998, our group firstly predicted the feasibility of a trans-catheter/ percutaneous approach adopting the EE concept [3]. Morales et al. described for the first time a device for beating heart EE repair with a tissue grasper [7]. Alfieri et al. [8] reported the early animal experience with a suture-based device for double-orifice repair with a beating-heart, via direct trans-atrial approach. The device had suction ports at its distal tip to grasp the leaflets under echo-guidance and subsequently approximate them by deploying two single sutures. Then the sutures were tied with a knot pusher to get the double orifice. In parallel, a percutaneous catheter called Mobius (Edwards Lifesciences, Irvine, California), with similar characteristics, had been developed [9]. The "Mobius" procedure involved a transeptal approach and the sequential grasping of the leaflets under echo-guidance. After needle penetration of the leaflets, the suture was exteriorized and fastened with a Nitinol suture clip to create the double orifice. The device proved safe and effective in the animal experience. Because suture-based approximation was closely replicating the surgical therapy, the device could be considered a "trans-catheter needle-holder." After the Milano II multicenter safety and feasibility trial, the program was discontinued for evidence of limited efficacy and durability. Webb et al. [10] reported the outcomes of 15 patients treated in four international sites: acute reduction of MR was obtained in 9 of 15 patients, but improvement in MR appeared durable in only 6 patients at 30 days. The main limitation for the success of the Mobius was lack of adequate image guidance (due to the poor echogenicity of the device). The limited durability was related to insufficient tissue penetration of the suture and to asymmetric deployment of sutures.

## 12.3   The Mitraclip: Clinical Evolution from First-in-Man to Commercial Use

The first animal report of the MitraClip is by St. Goar et al. in 2003 [11], who reported acute procedural success in 12 of 14 animals. Interestingly, in two animals the clip detached acutely from the anterior leaflet due to incomplete grasp. Today,

**Fig. 12.2** The MitraClip
percutaneous device

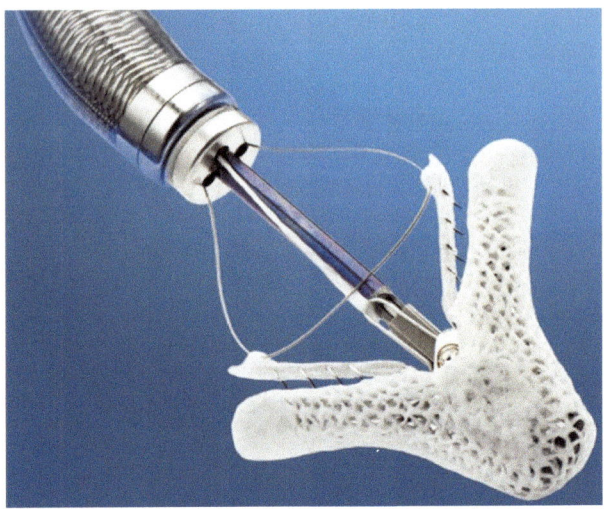

before final release, a careful analysis of leaflet incorporation into the clip is carried out to prevent clip detachment. Fann et al. [12] described the healing process in chronic animals implanted with the MitraClip, showing tissue incorporation of the device similar to that observed after surgical suture approximation [13].

The Mitraclip has been used in humans with success, due to the very promising animal experience. The main drivers for success of the therapy have been the precise and stable delivery system, the solid and reliable tissue approximation, the good visualization of the device, and its repositionability and retrievability. Although the MitraClip has been designed to replicate the surgical suture-based approach, tissue approximation is more efficient with better surface of coaptation, compared with suture. The main strength of the Mitraclip is feasibility of the procedure under beating heart conditions, guided directly by the position of the regurgitant jet. This is particularly valuable for functional MR. The main weakness is the limited applicability, according to strict anatomical features, whereas surgical EE can be applied more widely, mainly because of annuloplasty and combination with additional techniques. The MitraClip is a cobalt/chromium implant including two arms and two "grippers" independently securing the leaflets after grasping (Fig. 12.2). The clip arms and grippers are covered with polyester to enhance tissue healing. The implant is performed under general anesthesia and guided by 3-D TEE and fluoroscopy [14]. Transeptal puncture is performed in the mid-superior and posterior aspect of the fossa ovalis and symmetric implant is fundamental for effective and durable repair, similarly to the surgical technique. If the final result is unsatisfactory, the clip can be opened, inverted to release the leaflets and repositioned to obtain a double-orifice valve (Fig. 12.3). A second clip can be used to improve the result of the first one. The first-in-man procedure was performed in 2003, in a patient with anterior leaflet prolapse. Two years after the procedure, the patient showed mild residual MR and evidence of positive reverse remodeling [15].

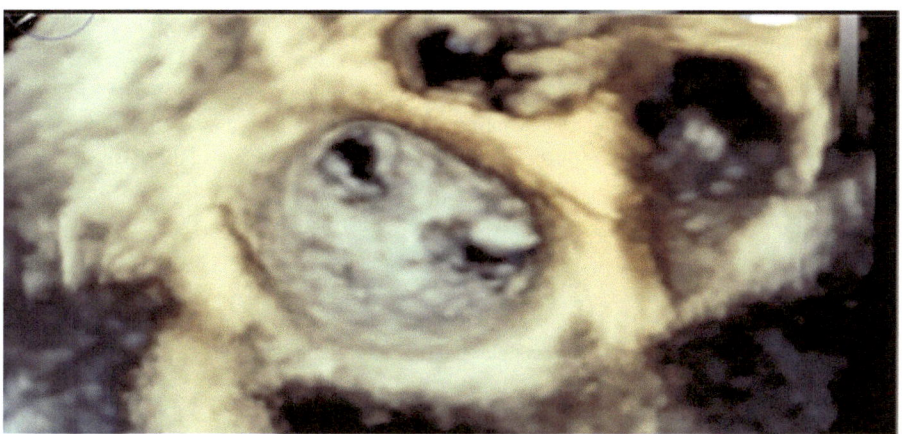

**Fig. 12.3** The MitraClip device implanted. A double-orifice valve is obtained during ventricular diastole at the 3-D trans-esophageal echocardiogram

## 12.4 Criteria and Indications for Patient Selection to Surgery or Percutaneous Treatment

Selection of the surgical versus percutaneous approach is challenging, in the absence of evidence. The decision is usually undertaken by a heart team and individualized on the basis of clinical and anatomical factors, keeping the surgical option as first choice. High-risk patients are considered for the procedure, but only a subgroup of patients can be treated by the MitraClip procedure, according to the anatomical criteria (Table 12.1) derived from the EVEREST inclusion protocol. In a quite likely future scenario, the combination of the MitraClip with an annuloplasty device could expand indications and improve efficacy and durability. Some patients treated with anatomical characteristics beyond the EVEREST criteria show reasonable short- and mid-term results [16, 17]. However, treating patients with more complex anatomy could be associated with procedural failure and shorter durability and should be performed only by expert operators. Surgical repair remains the gold standard in patients with degenerative MR being carried out with low risk and long-lasting results [18]. The Mitraclip procedure should be considered in inoperable or high risk patients due to advanced age and comorbidities. In degenerative MR, the ideal MitraClip candidate should have a prolapse or flail limited to one scallop. The width of the prolapsing segment should be less than 1.5 cm: larger flails are at risk of stenosis and require multiple clips. Technical feasibility is also influenced by the flail gap, a measure of the distance of the free edge of the prolapsing segment from the facing leaflet. For functional MR, the MitraClip is emerging as a valuable alternative [19], because surgical risk is usually higher [20], the survival benefit after surgery has not yet been demonstrated [21] and the repair is less durable [22]. Therefore, in presence of favorable anatomical characteristics, MitraClip represents a valid therapeutic option, unless the patient is a low-risk surgical candidate.

**Table 12.1** Echodoppler criteria for eligibility to the MitraClip therapy

| *Inclusion* |
| --- |
| Grade 3 to 4+ (moderate-severe to severe) MR |
| MR originating from the central 2/3 of the valve (A2-P2) |
| Degenerative or functional etiology |
| Sufficient tissue for mechanical capture of the valve |
| *Exclusion* |
| Rheumatic MR |
| MVA area <4 cm$^2$ |
| Flail gap >10 mm |
| Flail width >15 mm |
| LV systolic internal dimension >55 mm |
| LV ejection fraction <25 % |

Minimization of invasiveness and intraprocedural online assessment of the result are the main advantages of the MitraClip as compared with surgery. The main challenge remains the selection of the patients. It is mandatory that those challenges are overcome by a true teamwork effort, to enable a safe and effective introduction of the percutaneous techniques in clinical practice.

# References

1. Alfieri O, Maisano F, De Bonis M, et al. The double-orifice technique in mitral valve repair: a simple solution for complex problems. J Thorac Cardiovasc Surg. 2001;122:674–81.
2. Maisano F, Schreuder JJ, Oppizzi M, Fiorani B, Fino C, Alfieri O. The double-orifice technique as a standardized approach to treat mitral regurgitation due to severe myxomatous disease: surgical technique. Eur J Cardiothorac Surg. 2000;17:201–5.
3. Maisano F, Torracca L, Oppizzi M, et al. The edge-to-edge technique: a simplified method to correct mitral insufficiency. Eur J Cardiothorac Surg. 1998;13:240–5; discussion 245–6.
4. Gillinov AM, Cosgrove DM, Blackstone EH, et al. Durability of mitral valve repair for degenerative disease. J Thorac Cardiovasc Surg. 1998;116:734–43.
5. Maisano F, Caldarola A, Blasio A, De Bonis M, La Canna G, Alfieri O. Midterm results of edge-to-edge mitral valve repair without annuloplasty. J Thorac Cardiovasc Surg. 2003;126: 1987–97.
6. Maisano F, Vigano G, Blasio A, Colombo A, Calabrese C, Alfieri O. Surgical isolated edge-to-edge mitral valve repair without annuloplasty: clinical proof of the principle for an endovascular approach. EuroIntervention. 2006;2:181–6.
7. Morales DL, Madigan JD, Choudhri AF, et al. Development of an off bypass mitral valve repair. Heart Surg Forum. 1999;2:115–20.
8. Alfieri O, Elefteriades JA, Chapolini RJ, et al. Novel suture device for beating-heart mitral leaflet approximation. Ann Thorac Surg. 2002;74:1488–93.
9. Naqvi TZ, Buchbinder M, Zarbatany D, et al. Beating-heart percutaneous mitral valve repair using a transcatheter endovascular suturing device in an animal model. Catheter Cardiovasc Interv. 2007;69:525–31.
10. Webb JG, Maisano F, Vahanian A, et al. Percutaneous suture edge-to-edge repair of the mitral valve. EuroIntervention. 2009;5:86–9.
11. St Goar FG, Fann JI, Komtebedde J, et al. Endovascular edge-to-edge mitral valve repair: short-term results in a porcine model. Circulation. 2003;108:1990–3.

12. Fann JI, St Goar FG, Komtebedde J, et al. Beating heart catheterbased edge-to-edge mitral valve procedure in a porcine model: efficacy and healing response. Circulation. 2004;110: 988–93.
13. Privitera S, Butany J, Cusimano RJ, Silversides C, Ross H, Leask R. Images in cardiovascular medicine. Alfieri mitral valve repair: clinical outcome and pathology. Circulation. 2002;106: e173–4.
14. Swaans MJ, Van den Branden BJ, Van der Heyden JA, et al. Three-dimensional transoesopha-geal echocardiography in a patient undergoing percutaneous mitral valve repair using the edge-to-edge clip technique. Eur J Echocardiogr. 2009;10:982–3.
15. Condado JA, Acquatella H, Rodriguez L, Whitlow P, Velez-Gimo M, St Goar FG. Percutaneous edge-to-edge mitral valve repair: 2-year follow-up in the first human case. Catheter Cardiovasc Interv. 2006;67:323–5.
16. Tamburino C, Ussia GP, Maisano F, et al. Percutaneous mitral valve repair with the MitraClip system: acute results from a real world setting. Eur Heart J. 2010;31:1382–9.
17. Franzen O, Baldus S, Rudolph V, et al. Acute outcomes of MitraClip therapy for mitral regurgitation in high-surgical-risk patients: emphasis on adverse valve morphology and severe left ventricular dysfunction. Eur Heart J. 2010;31:1373–81.
18. Gammie JS, Sheng S, Griffith BP, et al. Trends in mitral valve surgery in the United States: results from the Society of Thoracic Surgeons Adult Cardiac Surgery Database. Ann Thorac Surg. 2009;87:1431–7; discussion 1437–9.
19. Taramasso M, Maisano F, Latib A, Denti P, Buzzatti N, Cioni M, La Canna G, Colombo A, Alfieri O. Clinical outcomes of MitraClip for the treatment of functional mitral regurgitation. EuroIntervention. 2014;10(6):746–52.
20. De Bonis M, Taramasso M, Grimaldi A, et al. The GeoForm annuloplasty ring for the surgical treatment of functional mitral regurgitation in advanced dilated cardiomyopathy. Eur J Cardiothorac Surg. 2011;40:488–95.
21. Wu AH, Aaronson KD, Bolling SF, Pagani FD, Welch K, Koelling TM. Impact of mitral valve annuloplasty on mortality risk in patients with mitral regurgitation and left ventricular systolic dysfunction. J Am Coll Cardiol. 2005;45:381–7.
22. Tahta SA, Oury JH, Maxwell JM, Hiro SP, Duran CM. Outcome after mitral valve repair for functional ischemic mitral regurgitation. J Heart Valve Dis. 2002;11:11–8; discussion 18–9.

# State of the Art of the MitraClip Therapy: Who, When, and How?

**13**

Paolo Denti, Nicola Buzzatti, and Giovanni La Canna

## 13.1 Introduction

Despite the poor prognosis associated with severe mitral regurgitation (MR) [1, 2] and the good results provided by surgical treatment [3, 4], approximately 50 % of the patients affected by severe MR remain untreated, mainly due to their advanced age and/or the presence of left ventricle dysfunction and comorbidities [5]. Transcatheter mitral therapies are currently emerging as an option to treat those high-risk or inoperable patients.

Thanks to its simplicity, the concept of surgical Alfieri's "edge-to-edge" technique [6], which approximates the two free edges of the mitral leaflets where coaptation is inadequate, has been widely borrowed by many of the transcatheter technologies that initially appeared on the scene.

Morales et al. first described a device for beating-heart edge-to-edge repair using a tissue grasper [7], while Alfieri et al. reported the preliminary animal experience with a suture-based device for edge-to-edge repair using a beating-heart direct transatrial approach [8]. This device had suction ports at its distal tip to grasp the leaflets under echo guidance and subsequently approximate them by deploying two single sutures. Then the sutures were tied with a knot pusher to obtain the double-orifice MV configuration. In parallel, the Mobius device (Edwards Lifesciences, Irvine, California), a percutaneous catheter with similar characteristics, had been developed [9]. The procedure was performed via a percutaneous transseptal approach and consisted in the sequential grasping of the leaflets under echo guidance, needle penetration of the leaflets, exteriorization, and fastening of the suture with a Nitinol clip. Since suture-based approximation was closely replicating the

P. Denti (✉) • N. Buzzatti • G. La Canna
Department of Cardiac Surgery, IRCCS San Raffaele University Hospital,
Via Olgettina, 60, Milan 20100, Italy
e-mail: paolodenti@hotmail.com; buzzatti.nicola@hsr.it; Lacanna.giovanni@hsr.it

© Springer International Publishing Switzerland 2015
O. Alfieri et al. (eds.), *Edge-to-Edge Mitral Repair: From a Surgical to a Percutaneous Approach*, DOI 10.1007/978-3-319-19893-4_13

137

surgical therapy, the device could be considered a "transcatheter needle holder." The device was proved to be safe and effective in animal setting, but after an initial first-in-man experience, the program was discontinued because of limited efficacy and durability. Webb et al. reported the results of 15 patients treated in 4 international sites [10]: initial reduction of MR was obtained in 9 of 15 patients, but improvement in MR appeared durable only in 6 patients after 30 days. The main limitation of the Mobius device was the lack of adequate image guidance due to the poor echogenicity of the system leading to insufficient tissue penetration and asymmetric deployment of the sutures, which were probably responsible for the limited durability of the repair.

The MitraClip System (Abbott Laboratories, Abbott Park, Illinois) has also been one of the first transcatheter techniques developed for percutaneous treatment of MR (the first case being performed in 2003 [11]), and it is the most used worldwide at present time, with approximately 20,000 procedures already performed. The technology has received CE mark in 2008 and is available for clinical use in Europe. It has been included in the ESC/EACTS Valvular Heart Disease Guidelines as a treatment option for high-risk and inoperable patients as decided after Heart Team discussion [12]. In the USA, FDA approval was achieved only for degenerative MR (DMR) in 2014, and the device still remains investigational for the treatment of functional MR (FMR).

## 13.2    The Procedure

The MitraClip delivery system is made up of a sophisticated triaxial catheter system (steerable guide catheter and clip delivery system catheter) and an implantable clip, available in one single size (Fig. 13.1). The clip delivery system, which can be steered in four directions, has the MitraClip device attached to its distal end; the guide catheter is 24 Fr at the level of the groin and 22 Fr at the atrial septum. The device is a cobalt-chromium implant with two arms and two "grippers" adjacent to

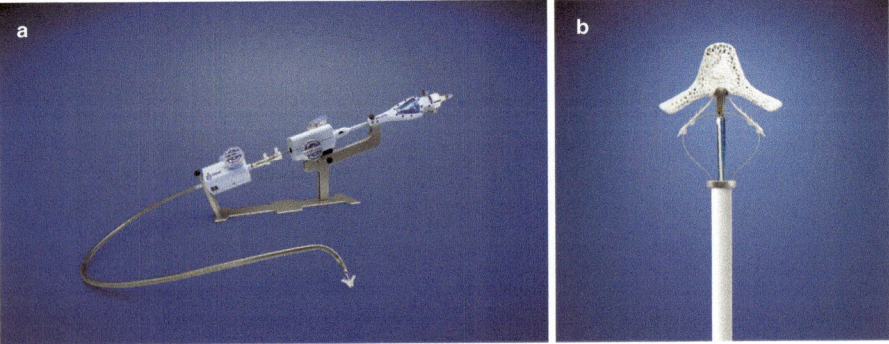

**Fig. 13.1** The MitraClip System: (**a**) the whole system including the delivery steerable catheter with the clip mounted and ready for implantation; (**b**) close up of the clip device

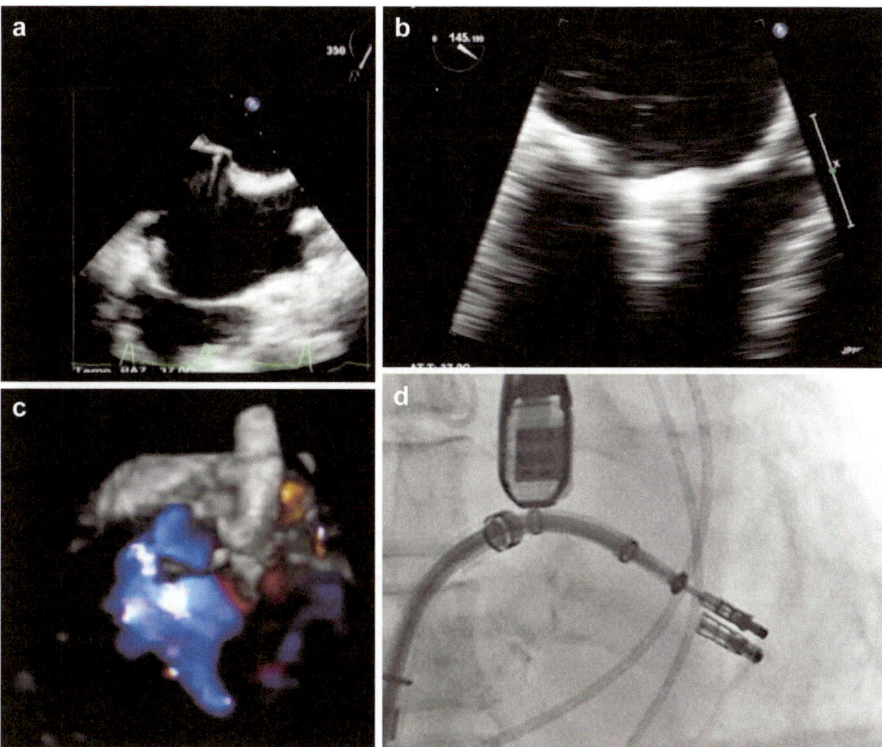

**Fig. 13.2** Subsequent steps of MitraClip procedure: (**a**) transseptal puncture; (**b**) leaflet grasping; (**c**) residual MR assessment after clip closure before clip detachment; (**d**) second clip positioning as seen in fluoroscopy

each arm to independently secure the leaflets following grasping. The clip arms and grippers are covered with polyester to enhance healing. The MitraClip is implanted through a sequence of standardized steps, under general anesthesia, guided by transesophageal echocardiography (TEE) and fluoroscopy. Currently, many procedures are performed under real-time 3D echocardiography with fusion imaging techniques, which makes them easier and more intuitive. After peripheral venous access at the groin, the atrial septum is crossed using diathermy in the mid-superior and posterior aspect of the fossa ovalis, to achieve proper alignment of the system (Fig. 13.2a); the location of the transseptal puncture is critical to reach the mitral valve leaflets with coaxial alignment to the long axis of the heart. Following transseptal puncture, a steerable guide catheter is advanced into the left atrium. Afterwards, the clip delivery system is inserted, and the MitraClip device is steered towards the mitral valve, at the origin of the regurgitant jet. The clip arms are opened and positioned perpendicularly to the line of coaptation; symmetric implantation is fundamental for an effective and durable repair, as in the setting of a surgical repair. The clip is advanced into the left ventricle and then retracted and partially closed to a "V" shape to engage the leaflets. Leaflets are grasped by gentle retraction of the clip towards the left atrium (Fig. 13.2b). To secure the leaflets into the device, the grippers are dropped and the clip is closed at approximately 60° to allow assessment of leaflet insertion. This step is reversible and resembles the surgical procedure, when a temporary central suture is used to assess symmetry and efficacy of the position. When the clip is closed, the final effect on MR reduction is evaluated using full-volume 3D color Doppler (Fig. 13.2c), and if the result of the implant is satisfactory, the clip is deployed. However, if necessary, at this stage the clip can still be reopened, inverted to release the leaflets, and repositioned. Alternatively a second clip can be used (Fig. 13.2d), but rarely more than two clips should be used in order to avoid mitral valve stenosis. Once the procedure is completed, percutaneous vascular closure is performed, and the patient is weaned from general anesthesia. Successful procedures have also been described under conscious sedation [13], although this has not become a routine approach, since good imaging guidance should not be traded off for less invasiveness.

## 13.3 Initial Results

The feasibility, safety, and efficacy of MitraClip repair were initially assessed by two subsequent studies, the EVEREST I [14] and II trials [15]; the latter compared percutaneous to conventional surgical repair in a randomized fashion. Data of this study showed a reduced rate of 30 days MACE in the MitraClip group compared to the surgical one (15 % vs 48 %, $p < 0.001$, although this was mainly driven by the transfusion rate), but a significantly worse degree of residual MR and higher need of mitral reintervention at 12 months in the percutaneous group (20 % vs 2 %, $p < 0.001$). The 4-year results of this study were recently published [16]: survival rates were similar between the two groups (17.4 % vs 17.8 %, $p = 0.914$) although residual MR and need of mitral reintervention were confirmed to be higher in the MitraClip group (24.8 % vs 5.5 %, $p < 0.001$).

One of the main issues with the EVEREST II randomized trial is that the enrolled patients, mostly low risk and affected by DMR, are significantly different from those who are commonly treated in the "real-world" daily practice. Several single-center and multicenter studies have been published over the last years reporting the outcomes of MitraClip therapy in real-world settings. Most of the patients (≈70 %) included in the EVEREST High-Risk [17], ACCESS-EU [18], TRAMI [19], and Pilot European Sentinel Registry [20] were affected by FMR in the contest of large ventricles with poor ejection fraction. The remaining patients, affected by DMR, were usually very old and affected by a wide burden of comorbidities (such as renal failure, chronic pulmonary disease, etc.). Therefore, all patients submitted to MitraClip therapy in those real-world registries were characterized by a high preoperative risk (mean logistic euroSCORE 23.0 % in the ACCESS-EU registry).

Despite that, the MitraClip showed an excellent safety profile with an acute mortality of 2–4 % in the different series. Safety is actually one of the major advantages of the MitraClip procedure, since a very low mortality was observed even in patients with extremely poor ventricle function and critically ill conditions [21] as well as in elderly patients [22].

In the above reported series, 1-year survival and freedom from MR 3 to 4+ were around 75–80 % and significant clinical improvement was also observed. In the ACCESS-EU registry, a NYHA functional class I–II was present in 71.4 % of the cases at 12 months, with an improvement in the Minnesota Living With the Heart Failure score from $41.6 \pm 18.9$ to $28.1 \pm 20.1$ ($p < 0.0001$) and in the 6-min walking test from 274 to 334 m ($p < 0.0001$).

Although the procedure requires some degree of experience, a stiff marked learning curve effect was not documented [23]. Moreover, the versatile edge-to-edge mechanism of action of the MitraClip System allows the effective treatment of a large variety of mitral pathologies, from functional asymmetric tethering to myxomatous commissural prolapse [24] to hypertrophic SAM-related regurgitation [25].

## 13.4 Patient Selection

The anatomical including criteria for the MitraClip procedure are assessed by transesophageal echocardiography and are still based on those initially proposed by the EVEREST team (Table 13.1). Although still useful as a guideline, these criteria are not considered strictly mandatory anymore: as a matter of fact, they do not seem to be clearly associated with acute or long-term results and are currently not respected in a vast proportion of patients. Nevertheless, up to one-third of the patients who are screened for MitraClip treatment do not receive it because of anatomical ineligibility [26].

Besides the mere numeric parameters used in the EVEREST Trial, careful echocardiographic and clinical evaluation are both essential to achieve satisfactory results. Specific anatomical factors, such as calcifications, leaflet clefts, multiple jets, significant annular dilatation, extreme left-ventricular dilatation, and severe leaflet tethering, are among the most important factors to be assessed by the transesophageal echocardiography before intervention. In addition, a comprehensive patient assessment should be performed, including the expected clinical and quality of life benefits, to avoid futile procedures in patients whose cardiac disease or comorbidities are too advanced and may not allow any further significant improvement.

According to current guidelines [12, 27], transcatheter mitral repair should be reserved to symptomatic patients with suitable anatomy who are judged to be

**Table 13.1** Anatomical selection criteria for MitraClip procedures

| Recommended criteria | Caution criteria |
| --- | --- |
| Coaptation length $\geq 2$ mm | Short posterior leaflet $< 8$ mm |
| Coaptation depth $< 11$ mm | Restricted posterior leaflet |
| Flail gap $< 10$ mm | Calcification in the grasping area |
| Flail width $< 15$ mm | Clefts in the jet area |
| Mitral valve area $\geq 4$ cm$^2$ | Multiple jets |
| Central jet (A2-P2 area) | |

high-risk or inoperable by the Heart Team and who have an expected survival of at least 12 months.

Functional MR represents a particularly appealing target for transcatheter mitral repair because, in this setting, surgery may have high procedural risk, due to the presence of severe left-ventricular dysfunction, suboptimal results in terms of recurrent MR [28, 29], and no clear survival benefit [30].

## 13.5  Open Issues

### 13.5.1 Survival

A clear survival benefit after MitraClip repair has not been properly demonstrated. Two randomized trials, the RESHAPE in Europe and the COAPT in the USA, are currently enrolling patients affected by FMR with the purpose to compare percutaneous mitral repair with the MitraClip System to optimal medical therapy. However, Swaans et al. have recently reported a retrospective comparison between the outcomes of 139 high-risk patients submitted to MitraClip procedures, 53 patients to surgery, and 59 patients to conservative medical treatment [31]. All etiologies, FMR (77 %), DMR (18 %), and mixed (5 %), were included; mean follow-up time in the MitraClip group was $1.7 \pm 1.1$ years. After 1-year follow-up, the transcatheter repair and surgery groups showed similar survival rates (85.8 % and 85.2 %, respectively), whereas only 67.7 % of patients treated conservatively survived. After weighting for propensity score and controlling for risk factors, both the transcatheter repair ($p = 0.006$) and surgical ($p = 0.014$) groups showed better survival than the conservatively treated group. On the other hand, the MitraClip and surgical groups did not differ in terms of survival rates ($p = 0.430$).

Given the high-risk (sometimes extreme-risk) profile of the patients usually submitted to transcatheter mitral repair, a survival benefit may be difficult to observe and demonstrate due to their frequently reduced life expectancy (associated with the advanced cardiac disease in the FMR and with the advanced age and comorbidities in the DMR setting). Therefore, it may be questionable whether symptoms and quality of life improvement are a better (and sufficient) endpoint in these particular subsets of patients.

Notably, a randomized trial comparing surgery and optimal medical therapy has never been conducted.

### 13.5.2 Residual MR

Up until now, residual MR after transcatheter mitral repair has been acceptable, considering the high-risk profile of the patients, but inferior compared to the worldwide surgical experience, especially in the DMR setting. Increasing evidence is recently emerging that residual and recurrent MR after MitraClip repair may impair long-term outcomes. In the first 100 patients of the Swiss registry [32], acute procedural success defined as residual MR$\leq$2+ ($p=0.0069$) and discharge MR grade ($p=0.03$) were significant predictors of survival. Paranskaya et al. reported residual MR grade to be associated with a worse 1-year composite endpoint outcome including death, rehospitalization, and reintervention ($p=0.001$) [33]. Puls et al. have also documented an association between acute procedural failure (residual MR 3 to 4+) and increased follow-up mortality ($p=0.02$) and heart failure rehospitalization ($p=0.01$) [34]. Again, in the DMR high-risk patients enrolled in the EVEREST Trial, patients with 3 to 4+ residual MR showed a 12-month survival of 52 % vs 80 % of patients with 2+ MR and 83 % of patients with 1+ MR ($p=0.02$); interestingly no significant difference was observed in regard to survival between patients with 2+ vs 1+ ($p=0.61$). More data and longer follow-up are needed to adequately assess the impact of residual 2+ MR after MitraClip repair. Patients with residual 2+ MR are a particularly interesting subset of patients, since they represent a vast proportion of all treated patients ($\approx$40 %), and in surgical experience, moderate residual MR, both functional and degenerative, has been associated with impaired long-term outcomes [35, 36].

The lack of annuloplasty, which has been an intrinsic feature of MitraClip repair until now, is one of the major concerns in terms of suboptimal efficacy and residual/recurrent MR, since ring absence is a well-known predictor of repair failure in the surgical arena [37]. The combined use of upcoming mitral transcatheter annuloplasty devices may help to improve the results of MitraClip edge-to-edge technique.

Partial clip detachment, which is one of the causes of recurrent MR, is usually mainly observed during the early phase after the procedure, before the first 12 months [16, 18]. The abolishment of residual valve prolapse, in addition to simple MR reduction, could help in reducing this kind of complication in the DMR setting.

### 13.5.3  Need of Future Mitral Reinterventions

Mitral valve healing process after implantation of a MitraClip has been described in several cases [38]. Surgical mitral repair vs replacement after MitraClip remains a debated topic. Mitral repair seems feasible in a number of patients and has been reported up to 18 months after the transcatheter procedure [39]. However, the number of clips implanted (>2), the time from the initial procedure, and the degree of leaflet tissue alteration influence the chance of effective repair.

Moreover, the intrinsic edge-to-edge feature of the MitraClip, especially in case of central implantation, is a major concern regarding the possibility of future transcatheter mitral valve implantation; it would seem theoretically unsafe due to the risk of leaflet rupture and of inadequate prosthesis expansion because of the small residual mitral valve area. No experience, however, has been reported in this setting yet.

---

**Conclusion**

Transcatheter edge-to-edge mitral repair with the MitraClip System is the more experienced technique to treat MR with a percutaneous approach. Despite the patients' high-risk profile, it has provided good results in terms of safety and symptoms improvement and it is a viable option to treat high-risk and inoperable symptomatic patients. Residual MR grade remains suboptimal and may impair long-term outcomes, although in the next future the use of combined techniques, such as leaflet edge-to-edge and annuloplasty (which would perfectly mimic the standard surgical technique), promises to improve efficacy and durability. Before expanding the indications to low- and intermediate-risk patients, a better efficacy profile and additional long-term follow-up of data are warranted.

# References

1. Ling LH, Enriquez-Sarano M, Seward JB, Tajik AJ, Schaff HV, Bailey KR, et al. Clinical outcome of mitral regurgitation due to flail leaflet. N Engl J Med. 1996;335:1417–23.
2. Grigioni F, Enriquez-Sarano M, Zehr KJ, Bailey KR, Tajik AJ. Ischemic mitral regurgitation: long-term outcome and prognostic implications with quantitative Doppler assessment. Circulation. 2001;103:1759–64.
3. Enriquez-Sarano M, Schaff HV, Orszulak TA, Tajik AJ, Bailey KR, Frye RL. Valve repair improves the outcome of surgery for mitral regurgitation. A multivariate analysis. Circulation. 1995;91:1022–8.
4. Braun J, de Veire NR, Klautz RJM, Versteegh MIM, Holman ER, Westenberg JJM, et al. Restrictive mitral annuloplasty cures ischemic mitral regurgitation and heart failure. Ann Thorac Surg. 2008;85:430–7.
5. Mirabel M, Iung B, Baron G, Messika-Zeitoun D, Detaint D, Vanoverschelde JL, et al. What are the characteristics of patients with severe, symptomatic, mitral regurgitation who are denied surgery? Eur Heart J. 2007;28:1358–65.
6. Alfieri O, Maisano F, De Bonis M, Stefano PL, Torracca L, Oppizzi M, et al. The double-orifice technique in mitral valve repair: a simple solution for complex problems. J Thorac Cardiovasc Surg. 2001;122:674–81.
7. Morales DL, Madigan JD, Choudhri AF, Williams MR, Helman DN, Elder JB, et al. Development of an off bypass mitral valve repair. Heart Surg Forum. 1999;2:115–20.
8. Alfieri O, Elefteriades JA, Chapolini RJ, Steckel R, Allen WJ, Reed SW, et al. Novel suture device for beating-heart mitral leaflet approximation. Ann Thorac Surg. 2002;74:1488–93.
9. Naqvi TZ, Buchbinder M, Zarbatany D, Logan J, Molloy M, Balke G, et al. Beating-heart percutaneous mitral valve repair using a transcatheter endovascular suturing device in an animal model. Catheter Cardiovasc Interv. 2007;69:525–31.
10. Webb JG, Maisano F, Vahanian A, Munt B, Naqvi TZ, Bonan R, et al. Percutaneous suture edge-to-edge repair of the mitral valve. EuroIntervention. 2009;5:86–9.
11. Condado JA, Acquatella H, Rodriguez L, Whitlow P, Velez-Gimo M, St Goar FG. Percutaneous edge-to-edge mitral valve repair: 2-year follow-up in the first human case. Catheter Cardio Inte. 2006;67:323–5.
12. Vahanian A, Alfieri O, Andreotti F, Antunes MJ, Baron-Esquivias G, Baumgartner H, et al. Guidelines on the management of valvular heart disease (version 2012): The Joint Task Force on the Management of Valvular Heart Disease of the European Society of Cardiology (ESC) and the European Association for Cardio-Thoracic Surgery (EACTS). Eur J Cardiothorac Surg. 2012;42:S1–44.
13. Ussia GP, Barbanti M, Tamburino C. Feasibility of Percutaneous Transcatheter Mitral Valve Repair With the MitraClip (R) System Using Conscious Sedation. Catheter Cardiovasc Interv. 2010;75:1137–40.
14. Feldman T, Wasserman HS, Herrmann HC, Gray W, Block PC, Whitlow P, et al. Percutaneous mitral valve repair using the edge-to-edge technique: Six-month results of the EVEREST phase I clinical trial. J Am Coll Cardiol. 2005;46:2134–40.

15. Feldman T, Foster E, Glower DG, Kar S, Rinaldi MJ, Fail PS, et al. Percutaneous Repair or Surgery for Mitral Regurgitation. N Engl J Med. 2011;364:1395–406.
16. Mauri L, Foster E, Glower DD, Apruzzese P, Massaro JM, Herrmann HC, et al. 4-year results of a randomized controlled trial of percutaneous repair versus surgery for mitral regurgitation. J Am Coll Cardiol. 2013;62:317–28.
17. Glower DD, Kar S, Trento A, Lim DS, Bajwa T, Quesada R, et al. Percutaneous mitral valve repair for mitral regurgitation in high-risk patients: results of the EVEREST II study. J Am Coll Cardiol. 2014;64:172–81.
18. Maisano F, Franzen O, Baldus S, Schafer U, Hausleiter J, Butter C, et al. Percutaneous mitral valve interventions in the real world: early and 1-year results from the ACCESS-EU, a prospective, multicenter, nonrandomized post-approval study of the MitraClip Therapy in Europe. J Am Coll Cardiol. 2013;62:1052–61.
19. Baldus S, Schillinger W, Franzen O, Bekeredjian R, Sievert H, Schofer J, et al. MitraClip therapy in daily clinical practice: initial results from the German transcatheter mitral valve interventions (TRAMI) registry. Eur J Heart Failure. 2012;14:1050–5.
20. Nickenig G, Estevez-Loureiro R, Franzen O, Tamburino C, Vanderheyden M, Luscher TF, et al. Percutaneous mitral valve edge-to-edge repair: in-hospital results and 1-year follow-up of 628 patients of the 2011–2012 pilot European sentinel registry. J Am Coll Cardiol. 2014;64:875–84.
21. Rudolph V, Huntgeburth M, von Bardeleben RS, Boekstegers P, Lubos E, Schillinger W, et al. Clinical outcome of critically ill, not fully recompensated, patients undergoing MitraClip therapy. Eur J Heart Failure. 2014;16(11):1223–9.
22. Schillinger W, Hunlich M, Baldus S, Ouarrak T, Boekstegers P, Hink U, et al. Acute outcomes after MitraClip therapy in highly aged patients: results from the German TRAnscatheter Mitral valve Interventions (TRAMI) Registry. EuroIntervention. 2013;9:84–90.
23. Ledwoch J, Franke J, Baldus S, Schillinger W, Bekeredjian R, Boekstegers P, et al. Impact of the learning curve on outcome after transcatheter mitral valve repair: results from the German Mitral Valve Registry. Clin Res Cardiol (Official J German Cardiac Society). 2014;103(11):930–7.
24. Estevez-Loureiro R, Franzen O, Winter R, Sondergaard L, Jacobsen P, Cheung G, et al. Echocardiographic and clinical outcomes of central versus noncentral percutaneous edge-to-edge repair of degenerative mitral regurgitation. J Am Coll Cardiol. 2013;62:2370–7.
25. Schafer U, Frerker C, Thielsen T, Schewel D, Bader R, Kuck KH, et al. Targeting systolic anterior motion and left ventricular outflow tract obstruction in hypertrophic obstructed cardiomyopathy with a MitraClip. EuroIntervention. 2014. [Epub ahead of print].
26. Grayburn PA, Roberts BJ, Aston S, Anwar A, Hebeler Jr RF, Brown DL, et al. Mechanism and severity of mitral regurgitation by transesophageal echocardiography in patients referred for percutaneous valve repair. Am J Cardiol. 2011;108:882–7.
27. Nishimura RA, Otto CM, Bonow RO, Carabello BA, Erwin 3rd JP, Guyton RA, et al. 2014 AHA/ACC Guideline for the Management of Patients With Valvular Heart Disease: A Report of the American College of Cardiology/American Heart Association Task Force on Practice Guidelines. Circulation. 2014;129(23):e521–643.
28. McGee EC, Gillinov AM, Blackstone EH, Rajeswaran J, Cohen G, Najam G, et al. Recurrent mitral regurgitation after annuloplasty for functional ischemic mitral regurgitation. J Thorac Cardiol Surg. 2004;128:916–24.
29. Hung J, Papakostas L, Tahta SA, Hardy BG, Bollen BA, Duran CM, et al. Mechanism of recurrent ischemic mitral regurgitation after annuloplasty – continued LV remodeling as a moving target. Circulation. 2004;110:Ii85–Ii90.
30. Wu AH, Aaronson KD, Bolling SF, Pagani FD, Welch K, Koelling TM. Impact of mitral valve annuloplasty on mortality risk in patients with mitral regurgitation and left ventricular systolic dysfunction. J Am Coll Cardiol. 2005;45:381–7.
31. Swaans MJ, Bakker AL, Alipour A, Post MC, Kelder JC, de Kroon TL, et al. Survival of transcatheter mitral valve repair compared with surgical and conservative treatment in high-surgical-risk patients. JACC Cardiovasc Interv. 2014;7:875–81.

32. Surder D, Pedrazzini G, Gaemperli O, Biaggi P, Felix C, Rufibach K, et al. Predictors for efficacy of percutaneous mitral valve repair using the MitraClip system: the results of the MitraSwiss registry. Heart. 2013;99:1034–40.
33. Paranskaya L, D'Ancona G, Bozdag-Turan I, Akin I, Kische S, Turan GR, et al. Residual mitral valve regurgitation after percutaneous mitral valve repair with the MitraClip(R) system is a risk factor for adverse one-year outcome. Catheter Cardiovasc Interv. 2013;81:609–17.
34. Puls M, Tichelbacker T, Bleckmann A, Hunlich M, von der Ehe K, Beuthner BE, et al. Failure of acute procedural success predicts adverse outcome after percutaneous edge-to-edge mitral valve repair with MitraClip. EuroIntervention. 2014;9:1407–17.
35. Fattouch K, Sampognaro R, Speziale G, Salardino M, Novo G, Caruso M, et al. Impact of moderate ischemic mitral regurgitation after isolated coronary artery bypass grafting. Ann Thorac Surg. 2010;90:1187–94.
36. De Bonis M, Lapenna E, Lorusso R, Buzzati N, Gelsomino S, Taramasso M, et al. Very long-term results (up to 17 years) with the double-orifice mitral valve repair combined with ring annuloplasty for degenerative mitral regurgitation. J Thorac Cardiovasc Surg. 2012;144(5):1019–24.
37. De Bonis M, Lapenna E, Maisano F, Barili F, La Canna G, Buzzatti N, et al. Long-term results (</=18 Years) of the edge-to-edge mitral valve repair without annuloplasty in degenerative mitral regurgitation: implications for the percutaneous approach. Circulation. 2014;130:S19–24.
38. Ladich E, Michaels MB, Jones RM, McDermott E, Coleman L, Komtebedde J, et al. Pathological healing response of explanted MitraClip devices. Circulation. 2011;123:1418–27.
39. Argenziano M, Skipper E, Heimansohn D, Letsou GV, Woo YJ, Kron I, et al. Surgical revision after percutaneous mitral repair with the MitraClip device. Ann Thorac Surg. 2010;89:72–80.

# Clinical Results of the Percutaneous Edge-to-Edge Repair: Lights and Shadows

# 14

Maurizio Taramasso, Alberto Pozzoli, and Antonio Colombo

Mitral regurgitation (MR) is the most frequent valvular heart disease in developed countries [1]. MR can be organic (resulting from primary anatomical alterations affecting the valve leaflets or subvalvular apparatus: primary MR) or functional (resulting from left ventricular (LV) remodeling processes causing papillary muscle dislocation and leaflet tethering, in the absence of structural abnormalities of the valve: secondary MR).

The natural history of severe MR is unfavorable (Fig. 14.1), leading to worsening LV failure, pulmonary hypertension, atrial fibrillation, and death [2].

The most common etiology of organic MR in Western countries is degenerative MR (DMR) due to leaflet tissue alteration known as myxomatous degeneration or fibroelastic deficiency, leading to mitral valve (MV) prolapse or flail [3].

Secondary MR is the consequence of LV dysfunction and dilation due to the maladaptive process in the context of a post-ischemic or idiopathic dilated cardiomyopathy.

Surgical repair represents the optimal treatment for severe DMR because of its well-documented advantages over valve replacement in terms of perioperative mortality, preservation of postoperative LV function, and long-term survival [4, 5].

M. Taramasso (✉)
Department of Cardiac Surgery, University Hospital Zurich,
Rämistrasse 100, Zurich 8091, Switzerland
e-mail: m.taramasso@gmail.com

A. Pozzoli
Department of Cardiac Surgery, IRCCS San Raffaele University Hospital,
Via Olgettina 60, Milan 20132, Italy
e-mail: albertopozzoli@gmail.com

A. Colombo
Department of Interventional Cardiology, IRCCS San Raffaele University Hospital,
Via Olgettina 60, Milan 20132, Italy

EMO-GVM Centro Cuore Columbus, Via M. Buonarroti 48, Milan 20132, Italy
e-mail: colombo@emocolumbus.it; antonio.colombo@hsr.it

© Springer International Publishing Switzerland 2015
O. Alfieri et al. (eds.), *Edge-to-Edge Mitral Repair: From a Surgical to a Percutaneous Approach*, DOI 10.1007/978-3-319-19893-4_14

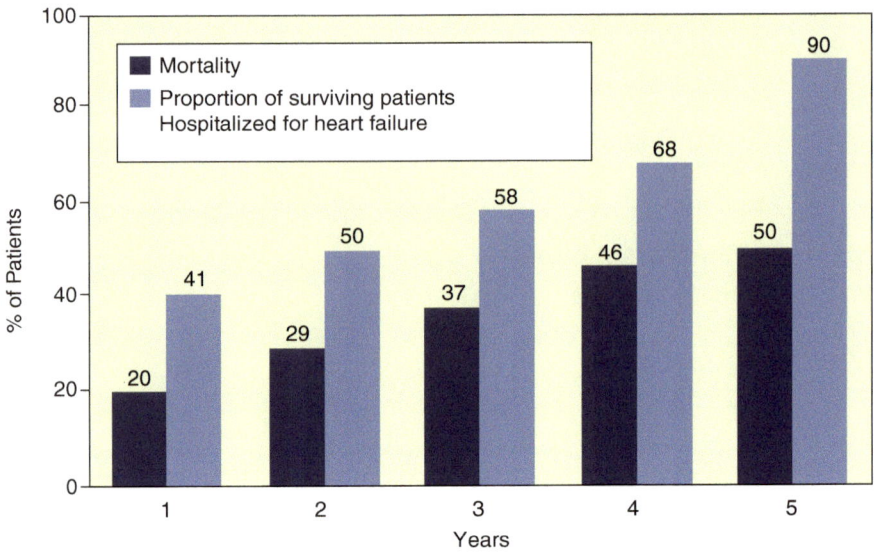

**Fig. 14.1** Mortality and rates of hospitalization for heart failure in unoperated patients with severe MR (Adapted from Goel et al. [39])

Indeed, if performed before the onset of limiting symptoms or the development of LV dysfunction, MV repair is able to restore normal life expectancy and quality of life [6]. By contrast, surgical correction of functional MR (FMR) is controversial, because the prognosis of the patient is more related to the cardiomyopathic process than to MR. Outcomes after surgical correction of FMR remain sub-optimal in many cases, and perioperative mortality is not negligible [7–10].

The Euro Heart Survey conducted by the European Society of Cardiology (ESC) showed that up to 50 % of patients with severe MR are today denied surgical treatment because they were felt to be at too high risk for surgery owing to advanced age or comorbidities [11]. Therefore, over the past few years, new trans-catheter techniques have been developed to treat MR with less invasive approaches. Different types of trans-catheter procedures are becoming available. Currently, the procedure with the widest clinical experience is the percutaneous edge-to-edge performed with the MitraClip System (Abbott Park, IL, USA) (Fig. 14.2).

The EVEREST study (*E*ndovascular *V*alve *E*dge-to-Edge *Re*pair of Mitral Regurgitation *St*udy) comprises a series of trials, including the first randomized controlled trial in which percutaneous treatment was compared with surgical treatment in selected patients with MR (mainly of degenerative etiology). The study results concluded that 1 year after the procedure, surgery was superior to percutaneous treatment in terms of efficacy whereas the percutaneous treatment was associated with higher safety. In a post hoc analysis, the MitraClip therapy has proven to be non-inferior to surgery in terms of effectiveness in three subgroups of patients: patients older than 70 years, those with LV dysfunction, and those with FMR [12–26].

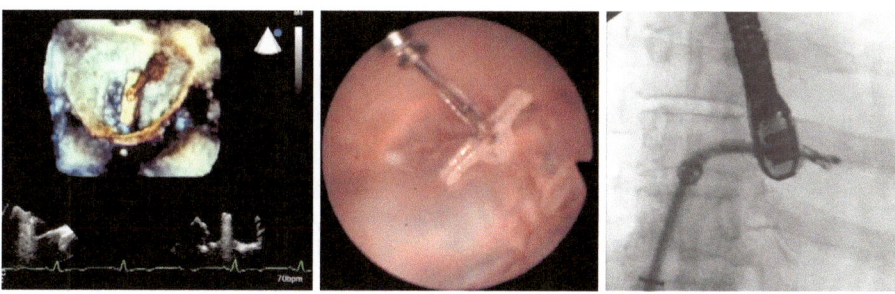

**Fig. 14.2** Trans-catheter edge-to-edge procedure with the MitraClip therapy

Primary and secondary MR are very different entities in terms of etiology, prognosis, and management and they will therefore be discussed separately in this chapter.

## 14.1 Degenerative Mitral Regurgitation

The only trans-catheter device that has been evaluated in organic MR is the MitraClip therapy. Currently, most patients undergoing the MitraClip procedure are non-surgical high-risk candidates. Data from the EVEREST trials and from registries in Europe and the USA suggest that the MitraClip technique has a procedural success rate (post-procedural MR ≤2+) of about 75 %, is relatively safe and generally well-tolerated, even by patients in poor clinical conditions [12–26]. According to the ESC 2012 VHD Guidelines [27], the percutaneous edge-to-edge procedure may be considered in patients with symptomatic severe DMR who fulfil the echocardiographic criteria of eligibility, are judged inoperable or at high surgical risk by a "Heart Team," and have a life expectancy greater than 1 year (class IIb, level of evidence C).

The High Risk Study (HRS), an arm of the EVEREST II trial, enrolled symptomatic patients with moderate to severe or severe MR for whom surgical perioperative risk of mortality was estimated to be higher than 12 %, using either the Society of Thoracic Surgeons (STS) calculator or surgeon coinvestigator estimated mortality risk of at least 12 % based on prespecified criteria. A degenerative etiology was present in 105 patients. Thirty-day mortality was 6.7 %. At 1 year, 85 % of the DMR patients had a reduction in MR; 87 % of the patients improved to a NYHA functional class I/II. The annual rate of hospitalization for heart failure was significantly reduced compared to baseline after MitraClip implantation [28].

The ACCESS-EU study is the first large database reporting outcomes of the MitraClip in a high-risk population of patients. The study had no pre-specified criteria for treatment and it provides a better reflection of the real-world practice: while most of the patients enrolled in the EVEREST trials were surgical candidates, the majority of the patients treated in the ACCESS-EU are high-risk surgical patients [29].

In the ACCESS-EU study, out of 567 patients undergoing the MitraClip procedure, 117 patients (20 %) had a DMR etiology [30]. The overall DMR cohort included elderly patients (75.6 ± 12.1 years) with 61.5 % of them over 75 years of age and 49.6 % male gender. The majority of ACCESS-EU Phase I DMR patients presented multiple co-morbidities at baseline. Approximately one quarter (23.9 %) of the patients had previous cardiovascular surgery including coronary artery bypass grafting (17.1 %) and 27.6 % of patients underwent percutaneous coronary intervention prior to enrolment in the ACCESS-EU study. The vast majority of patients (96.6 %) in the DMR cohort had a mitral regurgitation grade 3+ or 4+ at baseline and most (73.1 %) were symptomatic with NYHA Functional Class III or IV. Mean logEuroS-CORE I for the entire DMR cohort was 15.5 ± 13.3 %. Stratification into high- and low-risk patients revealed important demographic differences culminating in mean logEuroSCORE I of 33.1 ± 11.5 % and 8.6 ± 5.1 % for the two cohorts, respectively.

Procedural success was 94.9 %. Overall, mean length of stay in the intensive care unit (ICU), cardiac care unit (CCU), or post-anesthesia care unit (PACU) following the MitraClip procedure was 2.3 ± 2.6 days with a median of 1 day, with no differences between high-risk and low-risk DMR patients. However, the median post-procedural hospital stay was slightly longer for high–surgical risk patients when compared to low surgical risk patients (7.2 ± 4.3 days for high risk vs. 6.5 ± 5.5 days for low risk). Also, a significantly larger proportion of low risk patients were discharged home with or without home health care than high-risk patients (82.9 % and 74.2 % respectively, $p = 0.003$) [30].

About 90 % of patients achieved an MR reduction to grade ≤ 2+ at discharge, and 60 % achieved an MR reduction to grade ≤ 1+ at discharge.

Incidence of perioperative adverse events was low (stroke 0.9 %, myocardial infarction 0.9 %, acute renal failure 2.6 %, bleeding complication 3.4 %, mitral valve surgery 1.7 %). Thirty-day mortality was 6.0 % (9.1 % and 4.8 % for high- and low-risk subgroups, respectively). Causes of death were classified as cardiac in 42.9 %.

Overall rate of freedom from MR > grade 2+ was 75 % at 12 months. Meaningful clinical improvements were observed: 80.8 % of the patients were in NYHA functional class I–II at 1-year follow-up. Both Minnesota Living with Heart Failure questionnaire (MLHFQ) scores and 6MWT distance improved significantly at 12 months compared with baseline. Overall mortality at 1 year was 17 % [30].

The results of the ACCESS-EU DMR study showed that MitraClip therapy might serve as a complementary non-surgical therapeutic option for selected DMR patients who are considered at high risk or ineligible for surgery, providing significant reductions in MR and improvements in clinical outcomes at 12 months.

Lim et al. recently reported the mid-term results of 127 DMR patients with prohibitive surgical risk who underwent MitraClip treatment. "Prohibitive risk" included patients with a STS predicted risk of mortality for mitral valve replacement of ≥ 8 % or with factors for prohibitive surgical risk not included in the STS risk calculator. Patients were elderly (mean age 82 years), severely symptomatic (87 % NYHA Class III–IV), with an STS mortality score of 13.2 ± 7.3 %. MitraClip was successfully implanted in 95 % of the cases. Hospital stay was about 3 days. Thirty-days mortality was 6.3 %. Peri-procedural adverse events rate was low, including myocardial infarction in 0.8 %, stroke in 2.4 %, acute renal failure 1.6 %, major vascular complications in 5.5 % [31].

One-year mortality was 23.6 %. The majority of surviving patients (82.9 %) remained with MR $\leq$2+ at 1 year and 86.9 % were in NYHA Functional Class I–II. Left ventricular end-diastolic volume decreased ($125.1 \pm 40.1$ mL to $108.5 \pm 37.9$ mL, $p < 0.0001$). SF-36 quality-of-life scores improved and hospitalizations for heart failure were reduced in patients whose MR was reduced. The conclusions of the study are that MitraClip treatment in prohibitive surgical risk patients is associated with safety and good clinical outcomes, including rehospitalization decrease, functional improvements, and favorable ventricular remodeling at 1 year.

Good clinical outcomes in the setting of DMR elderly patients were reported by Taramasso et al. in a single center experience [32]. Forty-eight high-risk consecutive patients with severe DMR underwent MitraClip implantation (mean age 78.5 years; 57 % of the patients were older than 80 years). Mean STS score was 12 % and 71 % of patients were in New York Heart Association class III or IV. The device was successfully implanted in 47 of 48 patients (98 %). In-hospital mortality was very low (1/48 patients, 2 %). Perioperative major events included 2 % incidence of acute renal failure and 4 % of bleeding complication, while no cerebrovascular accident or acute myocardial infarction was reported. The median intensive care unit stay was 22 h. Pre-discharge echocardiography showed a mitral regurgitation reduction to grade 2+ or less in 43 of 47 patients (91.5 %). Actuarial survival was 89 % and 70.2 % at 1 and 2 years, respectively (82 % in patients aged <80 years and 95 % in patients older than 80 years at 1 year). Freedom from mitral regurgitation 3+ or greater was 80 % at 1 year and 76.6 % at 2 years. At 1 year, 93 % of survivors were in NYHA class I–II (100 % of patients aged <80 years and 88 % of patients aged $\geq$80 years). Significant quality of life and functional status improvements were documented at follow-up.

An improvement in perceived quality of life after MitraClip therapy for DMR was documented also by Ussia et al. [33] in a small series of 14 consecutive high risk patients with DMR who reported both physical and mental status improvement 6 months after the procedure.

In this scenario, trans-catheter edge-to-edge treatment of DMR could play a relevant clinical role in the near future. Several reports suggest that the reduction in invasiveness of the trans-catheter edge-to-edge is associated to low procedural risk and to significant clinical benefit, and this can be beneficial in the subset of very old and high-risk populations. This is particularly true in patients with associated cardiac conditions (i.e., associated coronary artery disease or atrial fibrillation), because trans-catheter interventions offer the unique opportunity of staging interventions to mitigate risk. For all these reasons the MitraClip procedure is now approved by the Federal Drug Administration (FDA) in patients with DMR considered at very high risk for surgical treatment.

## 14.2    Functional Mitral Regurgitation

The use of trans-catheter edge-to-edge to treat isolated FMR has exactly the same level of evidence and class of indication as the surgical treatment, reflecting a similar lack of evidence to support a more aggressive treatment strategy. In 2012, MitraClip was recommended by both the ESC Heart Failure and ESC/EACTS guidelines on valvular heart disease [27] for patients with symptomatic severe secondary MR despite optimal medical therapy (including CRT if indicated), with anatomical suitability, who are judged inoperable or at high surgical risk by a team of cardiologists and cardiac surgeons, and with a life expectancy greater than 1 year (recommendation class IIb, level of evidence C).

MitraClip therapy has been performed to treat FMR in high-risk and end-stage patients with favorable safety and efficacy results. Several clinical experiences with satisfactory acute and midterm results in FMR are now reported in the literature.

The High-Risk Registry of the EVEREST II study is the first to suggest a potential prognostic benefit in high-risk patients treated with the MitraClip in both the degenerative and functional MR groups. Patients treated with the MitraClip had a better survival rate at 1 year compared to a matched group managed with optimal medical treatment alone. In addition, the registry demonstrated a significant reduction in heart failure hospitalization by a factor of approximately 50 % as compared to the year before implantation, improvement in clinical symptoms, and significant LV reverse remodeling over 12 months in patients submitted to MitraClip therapy [28].

The ACCESS-EU registry [29] offers a snapshot of the characteristics of patients who currently undergo the procedure in the European post-market real word: they are mainly elderly patients with comorbidities, with high surgical risk profile or who are inoperable, and with a high prevalence of FMR (more than 70 % of the total). The reported mortality at 30 days was 3.4 %, which is notably low, especially if we consider that the majority of patients were at high surgical risk (Logistic EuroSCORE I $23 \pm 18$ %) and affected by FMR secondary to chronic heart failure.

At 12 months, the survival rate was 82 %, and 79 % of patients showed a residual MR less than or equal to 2+. Although this degree of reduction is lower than that observed after surgical repair, the persistence of an MR grade less than or equal to mild-to-moderate could be a reasonable therapeutic target in patients at high surgical risk. Moreover, the ACCESS registry demonstrated a remarkable clinical effectiveness: 1 year after the procedure, 71 % of patients were in NYHA functional class I or II and most patients had an improvement in quality of life and a gain in functional capacity.

Satisfactory clinical results have also been reported by the German TRAnscatheter MItral valve interventions (TRAMI) registry [34] that enrolled 1,064 patients (525 patients $\geq$76 years and 539 patients <76 years; more than 70 % with FMR). Age was the most frequent reason for non-surgical treatment in the elderly. The in-hospital MACCE (death, myocardial infarction, stroke) was low in both groups (3.5 % vs. 3.4 %) and the proportion of non-severe mitral regurgitation at discharge was similar (95.8 % vs. 96.4 %, $p = 0.73$). A logistic regression model did not reveal any significant impact of age on acute efficacy and safety of MitraClip therapy, showing that elderly and younger patients have similar clinical benefits.

The Transcatheter Valve Treatment Sentinel Pilot Registry [35], a prospective, independent, consecutive collection of individual patient data, enrolled a total of 628 patients (mean age $74.2 \pm 9.7$ years) who underwent trans-catheter edge-to-edge between January 2011 and December 2012 in 25 centers in 8 European countries. The prevalent pathogenesis was functional mitral regurgitation (FMR) (72.0 %). The majority of patients (85.5 %) were highly symptomatic (New York Heart Association functional class III or higher), with a high logistic EuroSCORE I ($20.4 \pm 16.7$ %). Acute procedural success was high (95.4 %) and similar in FMR and degenerative mitral regurgitation. In-hospital mortality was low (2.9 %) and the estimated 1-year mortality was 15.3 %, which was similar for FMR and degenerative mitral regurgitation. The estimated 1-year rate of rehospitalization because of heart failure was 22.8 %. Paired echocardiographic data from the 1-year follow-up, available for 368 consecutive patients, showed a persistent reduction in the degree of mitral regurgitation at 1 year, with 6.0 % of patients with severe mitral regurgitation.

MitraClip therapy has been demonstrated to be feasible and safe even in critically ill patients (NYHA IV), leading to symptomatic improvement in over two-thirds of these patients; however, it is associated with an elevated 30-day mortality, compared to stable clinical conditions [36].

## 14.3 Other Applications

Even if it is a niche application, it is important to mention that the trans-catheter edge-to-edge has been recently used to successfully address LVOT obstruction due to mitral systolic anterior motion (SAM) in the context of HOCM, showing that SAM-induced obstruction might be a valuable target for the MitraClip [37].

Other settings are treatment of severe mitral regurgitation in the context of acute myocardial infarction [38].

### Conclusions

Although surgical repair remains the gold standard therapy, trans-catheter edge-to-edge treatment of DMR could play a relevant clinical role in the near future, especially in the subset of the very old and high-risk population.

Regarding FMR, now that the safety of the percutaneous edge-to-edge has been proved, MitraClip is considered as an alternative option for patients at high surgical risk. Some issues regarding efficacy and long-term durability have to be addressed in order to reduce the threshold of risk and expand Mitraclip therapy to lower risk population. Final results of the EVEREST II trial showed that when acute optimal results are achieved with MitraClip, durability up to 5 years is usually obtained. MitraClip therapy is not so far a palliative therapy, when properly performed. This implies correct patient selection and timing, advanced procedural imaging, and optimal procedural performance.

We need randomized data to confirm that the correction of FMR in patients with advanced LV dysfunction and significant MR does in fact result in a meaningful clinical impact. It may be that MitraClip therapy could allow patients at high surgical risk to be treated with acceptable safety and procedural outcomes, but whether this truly benefits patients as opposed to optimal medical therapy remains to be proven. The COAPT trial will randomize high-surgical-risk subjects with clinically significant FMR to MitraClip therapy plus optimal medical therapy versus optimal medical therapy alone

In the coming years, MitraClip has probably the potential to become a first-line option in patients with isolated FMR. Surgery will still be considered in intermediate risk patients, particularly when associate conditions (such as atrial fibrillation and coronary artery disease) are present.

However, we need to treat patients at an earlier stage, if we look for a significant prognostic benefit and in this context a heart team approach will be mandatory.

# References

1. Nkomo VT, et al. Burden of valvular heart diseases: a population-based study. Lancet. 2006;368:1005–11.
2. Ling LH, et al. Clinical outcome of mitral regurgitation due to flail leaflet. N Engl J Med. 1996;335:1417–23.
3. Anyanwu AC, Adams DH. Etiologic classification of degenerative mitral valve disease: Barlow's disease and fibroelastic deficiency. Semin Thorac Cardiovasc Surg. 2007;19:90–6.
4. Yun KL, Miller DC. Mitral valve repair versus replacement. Cardiol Clin. 1991;9:315–27.
5. Olson LJ, Subramanian R, Ackermann DM, et al. Surgical pathology of the mitral valve: a study of 712 cases spanning 21 years. Mayo Clin Proc. 1987;62:22–34.
6. Detaint D, et al. Surgical correction of mitral regurgitation in the elderly: outcomes and recent improvements. Circulation. 2006;114:265–72.
7. Kang DH, Kim MJ, Kang SJ, et al. Mitral valve repair versus revascularization alone in the treatment of ischemic mitral regurgitation. Circulation. 2006;114:I499–503.
8. Braun J, Bax JJ, Versteegh MI, et al. Preoperative left ventricular dimensions predict reverse remodeling following restrictive mitral annuloplasty in ischemic mitral regurgitation. Eur J Cardiothorac Surg. 2005;27:847–53.
9. Crabtree TD, Bailey MS, Moon MR, et al. Recurrent mitral regurgitation and risk factors for early and late mortality after mitral valve repair for functional ischemic mitral regurgitation. Ann Thorac Surg. 2008;85:1537–42.
10. De Bonis M, Taramasso M, Grimaldi A, et al. The GeoForm annuloplasty ring for the surgical treatment of functional mitral regurgitation in advanced dilated cardiomyopathy. Eur J Cardiothorac Surg. 2011;40:488–95.
11. Mirabel M, Iung B, Baron G, et al. What are the characteristics of patients with severe, symptomatic, mitral regurgitation who are denied surgery? Eur Heart J. 2007;28:1358–65.
12. Argenziano M, Skipper E, Heimansohn D, et al. Surgical revision after percutaneous mitral repair with the MitraClip device. Ann Thorac Surg. 2010;89:72–80.
13. Feldman T, Foster E, Glower DD, et al. Percutaneous repair or surgery for mitral regurgitation. N Engl J Med. 2011;364:1395–406.
14. Feldman T, Kar S, Rinaldi M, et al. Percutaneous mitral repair with the MitraClip system safety and midterm durability in the initial EVEREST (Endovascular Valve Edge-to-Edge REpair Study) cohort. J Am Coll Cardiol. 2009;54:686–94.
15. Feldman T, Wasserman HS, Herrmann HC, et al. Percutaneous mitral valve repair using the edge-to-edge technique: six-month results of the EVEREST phase I clinical trial. J Am Coll Cardiol. 2005;46:2134–40.

16. George JC, Varghese V, Dangas G, Feldman TE. Percutaneous mitral valve repair: lessons from the EVEREST II (Endovascular Valve Edge-to-Edge REpair Study) and beyond. JACC Cardiovasc Interv. 2011;4:825–7.

17. Glower D, Ailawadi G, Argenziano M, et al. EVEREST II randomized clinical trial: predictors of mitral valve replacement in de novo surgery or after the MitraClip procedure. J Thorac Cardiovasc Surg. 2012;143:S60–3.

18. Goldberg SL, Feldman T. Percutaneous mitral valve interventions: overview of new approaches. Curr Cardiol Rep. 2010;12:404–12.

19. Herrmann HC, Gertz ZM, Silvestry FE, et al. Effects of atrial fibrillation on treatment of mitral regurgitation in the EVEREST II (Endovascular Valve Edge-to-Edge Repair Study) randomized trial. J Am Coll Cardiol. 2012;59:1312–9.

20. Herrmann HC, Kar S, Siegel R, et al. Effect of percutaneous mitral repair with the MitraClip (R) device on mitral valve area and gradient. EuroIntervention. 2009;4:437–42.

21. Herrmann HC, Rohatgi S, Wasserman HS, et al. Mitral valve hemodynamic effects of percutaneous edge-to-edge repair with the MitraClip™ device for mitral regurgitation. Catheter Cardiovasc Interv. 2006;68:821–8.

22. Ladich E, Michaels MB, Jones RM, et al. Pathological healing response of explanted MitraClip devices. Circulation. 2011;123:1418–27.

23. Mauri L, Garg P, Massaro JM, et al. The EVEREST II Trial: design and rationale for a randomized study of the evalve mitraclip system compared with mitral valve surgery for mitral regurgitation. Am Heart J. 2010;160:23–9.

24. Siegel RJ, Biner S, Rafique AM, et al. The acute hemodynamic effects of MitraClip therapy. J Am Coll Cardiol. 2011;57:1658–65.

25. Silvestry FE, Rodriguez LL, Herrmann HC, et al. Echocardiographic guidance and assessment of percutaneous repair for mitral regurgitation with the evalve MitraClip: lessons learned from EVEREST I. J Am Soc Echocardiogr. 2007;20:1131–40.

26. Whitlow PL, Feldman T, Pedersen WR, et al. Acute and 12-month results with catheter-based mitral valve leaflet repair: the EVEREST II (Endovascular Valve Edge-to-Edge Repair) high risk study. J Am Coll Cardiol. 2012;59:130–9.

27. Joint Task Force on the Management of Valvular Heart Disease of the European Society of Cardiology (ESC), European Association for Cardio-Thoracic Surgery (EACTS), Vahanian A, et al. Guidelines on the management of valvular heart disease (version 2012). Eur Heart J. 2012;33:2451–96.

28. Glower DD, Kar S, Trento A, et al. Percutaneous mitral valve repair for mitral regurgitation in high-risk patients: results of the EVEREST II study. J Am Coll Cardiol. 2014;64:172–81.

29. Maisano F, Franzen O, Baldus S, et al. Percutaneous mitral valve interventions in the real world: early and 1-year results from the ACCESS-EU, a prospective, multicenter, nonrandomized post-approval study of the MitraClip therapy in Europe. J Am Coll Cardiol. 2013;62:1052–61.

30. Reichenspurner H, Schillinger W, Baldus S, et al. Clinical outcomes through 12 months in patients with degenerative mitral regurgitation treated with the MitraClip® device in the ACCESS-EUrope Phase I trial. Eur J Cardiothorac Surg. 2013;44:e280–8.

31. Lim DS, Reynolds MR, Feldman T, et al. Improved functional status and quality of life in prohibitive surgical risk patients with degenerative mitral regurgitation after transcatheter mitral valve repair. J Am Coll Cardiol. 2014;64:182–92.

32. Taramasso M, Maisano F, Denti P, et al. Percutaneous edge-to-edge repair in high-risk and elderly patients with degenerative mitral regurgitation: midterm outcomes in a single-center experience. J Thorac Cardiovasc Surg. 2014;148:2743–50.

33. Ussia GP, Cammalleri V, Sarkar K, et al. Quality of life following percutaneous mitral valve repair with the MitraClip System. Int J Cardiol. 2012;155:194–200.

34. Schillinger W, Hünlich M, Baldus S, et al. Acute outcomes after MitraClip therapy in highly aged patients: results from the German TRAnscatheter Mitral valve Interventions (TRAMI) Registry. EuroIntervention. 2013;9:84–90.

35. Nickenig G, Estevez-Loureiro R, Franzen O, et al. Percutaneous mitral valve edge-to-edge repair: in-hospital results and 1-year follow-up of 628 patients of the 2011–2012 Pilot European Sentinel Registry. J Am Coll Cardiol. 2014;64:875–84.
36. Rudolph V, Huntgeburth M, von Bardeleben RS, et al. Clinical outcome of critically ill, not fully recompensated, patients undergoing MitraClip therapy. Eur J Heart Fail. 2014;16: 1223–9.
37. Schäfer U, Frerker C, Thielsen T, et al. Targeting systolic anterior motion and left ventricular outflow tract obstruction in hypertrophic obstructed cardiomyopathy with a MitraClip. EuroIntervention. 2014. pii: 20130310–02.
38. Bilge M, Alemdar R, Yasar AS. Successful percutaneous mitral valve repair with the MitraClip system of acute mitral regurgitation due to papillary muscle rupture as complication of acute myocardial infarction. Catheter Cardiovasc Interv. 2014;83:E137–40.
39. Goel SS, Bajaj N, Aggarwal B, et al. Prevalence and outcomes of unoperated patients with severe symptomatic mitral regurgitation and heart failure: comprehensive analysis to determine the potential role of MitraClip for this unmet need. J Am Coll Cardiol. 2014;63(2):185–6.

# Future Perspectives of the Edge-to-Edge Repair

**15**

Paolo Denti, Nicola Buzzatti, and Francesco Maisano

## 15.1 Introduction

Mitral regurgitation (MR) is a growing problem in the western world, due to the increasing prevalence of heart failure and population aging, since severe MR is known to be significantly associated with both these factors [1, 2]. The edge-to-edge (EE) technique as treatment of severe MR has by now demonstrated to have excellent long-term results and is considered a well-established and standard surgical technique. On the other hand, however, for the same reasons mentioned above, patients also tend to be at higher risk, on the average being older, and affected by more comorbidities and by more ventricular dysfunctions; for these reason, they are frequently excluded from intervention [3].

Although a number of transcatheter devices have emerged in the recent years to fill the gap of this unmet need [4], many of these technologies failed to prove feasibility, efficacy, and reliability and have been therefore discontinued. The first transcatheter technology to emerge as a reliable option, the MitraClip system, used the EE concept to target the mitral leaflet [5]. Today the MitraClip, with around 20,000 procedures performed worldwide, represents the most important experience in the field of percutaneous mitral repair. It has already received the CE mark in Europe and the FDA approval in the USA and is included in the

P. Denti (✉) • N. Buzzatti
Department of Cardiac Surgery, IRCCS San Raffaele University Hospital,
Via Olgettina, 60, Milan 20100, Italy
e-mail: buzzatti.nicola@hsr.it

F. Maisano
Cardiovascular Surgery Clinic, Herzzentrum, UniversitätsSpital Zürich,
Rämistrasse 71, Zürich 8006, Switzerland
e-mail: francesco.maisano@usz.ch

© Springer International Publishing Switzerland 2015
O. Alfieri et al. (eds.), *Edge-to-Edge Mitral Repair: From a Surgical to a Percutaneous Approach*, DOI 10.1007/978-3-319-19893-4_15

guidelines since 2012 [6]. Indeed, despite the high-risk profile of the treated patients, MitraClip has proved to yield good results in terms of safety, MR decrease, and symptoms improvement [7, 8].

## 15.2   Edge-to-Edge Devices Evolution

The *MitraClip* system is a unique and versatile technique. The procedure and device have not changed significantly over the years since its initial development and major future developments are difficult to predict.

Other transcatheter EE mitral repair devices have also been recently proposed, such as the *MitraFlex* device (TransCardiac Therapeutics, Atlanta, USA), which is still undergoing preclinical testing. Interestingly, it uses a combined approach: via a thoracoscopic transapical route, it deploys to the mitral leaflets a clip that is also attached to an artificial cord, which is in turn anchored in the inner LV myocardium.

A different concept, but somehow similar to the classic EE, is the one used by the *Percu-Pro* (Cardiosolutions, Stoughton, USA): it is a "buoy" that is anchored at the LV apex through a transseptal approach. This device acts as a spacer across the valve orifice providing a surface against which the leaflets can coapt. It is undergoing phase 1 trial and could be applied to both degenerative and functional MR. Open issues are the possible formation of thrombus on the device and the possibility of iatrogenic mitral stenosis. In addition, durability of the inflatable device needs to be investigated, as well as the consequences of chronic impact of the leaflets on the device.

Of note, EE is to be currently considered a contraindication to future mitral prosthesis implantation, so its use in case of anticipated need of such a subsequent procedure should be carefully evaluated.

## 15.3   Other Leaflet Procedures

In the next future, the transcatheter edge-to-edge technique will face other competitor technologies targeting the leaflets that have been proposed in the past few years. The most promising and rapidly spreading is the chordal implantation [9]. The main concept is to implant a chord, with various techniques, at the leaflet edge and anchor it to the left ventricle wall. The length of the NeoChord is adjusted real-time under echocardiographic guidance to reach optimal leaflet coaptation and MR reduction. Although most of current procedures are performed through a transapical access, a complete percutaneous approach is also under development. As its surgical equivalent, compared to the EE technique, chordal implantation has the theoretical advantage of respecting the natural mitral anatomy and physiology, with no risk of stenosis and no future obstacle of mitral valve prosthesis implantation. Again, as in the surgical setting, chordal repair will only be useful for DMR treatment with leaflet prolapse or flail, whereas the edge-to-edge remains far more versatile being able to treat basically all MR pathology including the FMR.

Notably, as in open surgery, the transcatheter edge-to-edge and chordal repair are not mutually exclusive but can be used together. Specifically, in surgical experience, the edge-to-edge has already proved excellent results when used as a "rescue" procedure in case of failure of other previously used mitral repair techniques [10].

## 15.4  Annuloplasty

Besides the leaflet procedure per se, what is really needed as the step forward to any transcatheter mitral repair technology is the addition of annuloplasty.

Annuloplasty is a fundamental step in every surgical mitral valve repair procedure. Its basic principle is to reduce the annular area restoring its normal ratio with the leaflet surface area. This leads to improved leaflet coaptation, decreased leaflet stress (which in turn avoids leaflet tear and suture dehiscence), and avoidance of progression of annular dilatation over time. A number of different surgical rings have been developed over the years to optimize these endpoints. The most recent rings are now cause-specific and geometrically shaped to accommodate different underlying pathologies [11].

In DMR, annuloplasty is always combined to a leaflet procedure. Flexible complete or incomplete rings are implanted whenever possible, since ring absence is a well-demonstrated factor associated with poor long-term outcomes [12, 13]. Specifically, long-term results of the EE technique without ring implantation reported a freedom from $MR \geq 3+$ at 12 years of $43 \pm 7.6$ % (Fig. 15.1), which raised to $64 \pm 7.6$ % in patients with acute optimal result (MR $\leq 1+$) [14]. By comparison the data from the same group of patients treated with combined EE and annuloplasty showed a freedom from $MR \geq 3+$ $83.8 \pm 3.4$ % at 14 years [15].

In FMR, undersized ring annuloplasty still represents the gold standard surgical treatment. In this setting, besides a careful preoperative anatomical selection, complete rigid rings are necessary to achieve effective and durable results [16, 17]. Reduction of the septolateral distance has a key role in correcting FMR [18, 19] and has therefore become a major target for modern geometrically shaped rings [20].

Different transcatheter annuloplasty devices have been proposed over the years to address MR.

The most currently promising technologies are the so-called direct annuloplasties.

The *Cardioband* (Valtech Cardio Inc., Or Yehuda, Israel, Fig. 15.2a) is a surgical Dacron band which can be implanted percutaneously [21]. Through a transseptal approach, the band is anchored to the atrial side of the mitral annulus via multiple helical anchors, from trigone to trigone. After delivery, the ring is adjusted "live" until adequate leaflet coaptation and MR reduction are achieved. The Cardioband is currently in clinical CE mark trial with promising results.

The *Mitralign* (Mitralign Inc., Tewksbury, MA USA, Fig. 15.2b) is a suturing plicating system, originally designed to plicate the mitral annulus at P1 and P3 levels from a retrograde ventricular approach [22]. Multiple plicating pledgets can be implanted along the annulus and interestingly, since the Mitralign is a true suturing system, different application of its suturing ability may be speculated. Mitralign CE

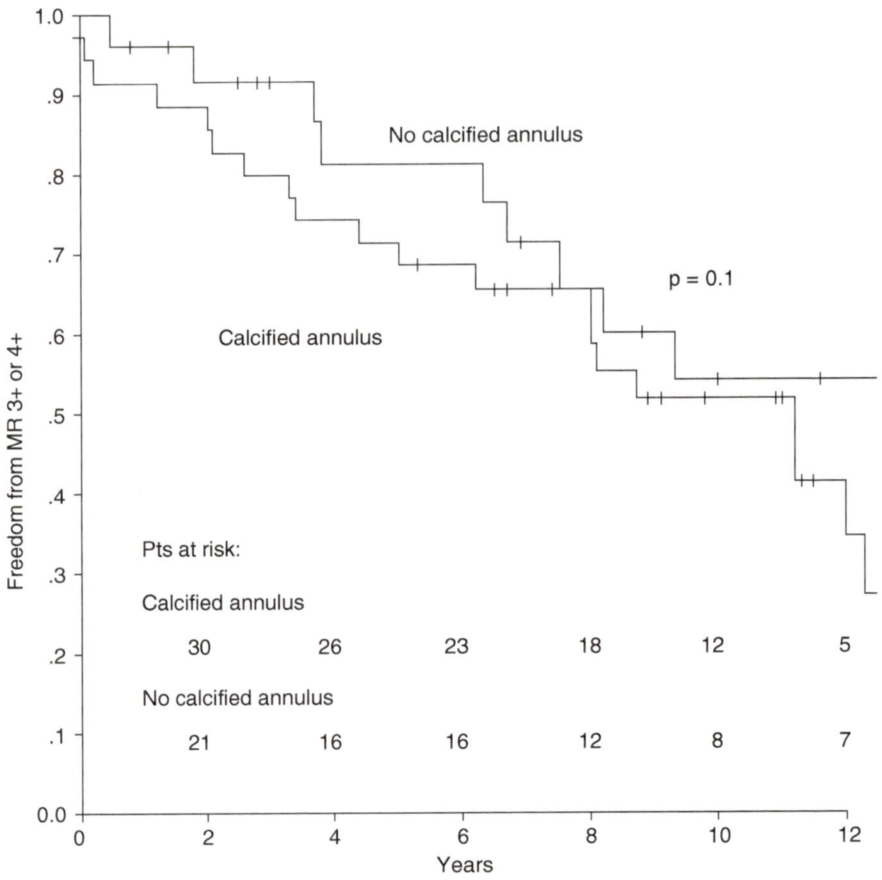

**Fig. 15.1** Freedom from MR recurrence 3 to 4+ in patients submitted to surgical edge-to-edge without ring implantation [14]

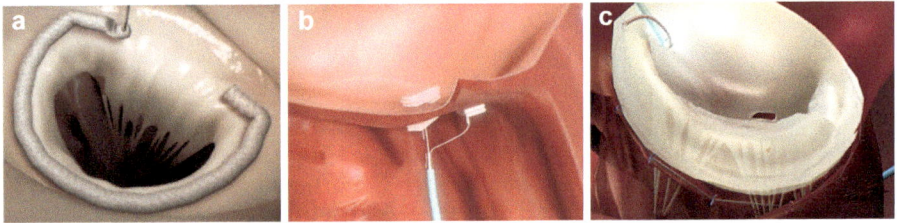

**Fig. 15.2** Direct mitral annuloplasty devices. (**a**) Cardioband; (**b**) Mitralign; (**c**) Accucinch

mark study on 61 patients has been already completed, and CE mark approval is expected in 2015.

The *Accucinch* (Guided Delivery System Inc., Santa Clara, CA, USA, Fig. 15.2c) also uses a retrograde ventricular approach to implant a series of anchors beneath the mitral annulus in the basal ventricular myocardium and connect them with a nitinol wire that is then used to cinch the mitral annulus and the basal ventricular wall. The Accucinch is currently under clinical evaluation.

A different major category of transcatheter mitral annuloplasty devices is the indirect coronary sinus system, which was actually the first to be developed and reach clinical application. These devices apply tension on the coronary sinus to indirectly reduce the mitral annulus dimension. Unfortunately this approach has shown to have serious limitations mainly due to the variable distance between the coronary sinus and the mitral annulus which significantly impair procedural efficacy [23] and due to the high risk of coronary artery compression.

For these reasons, coronary sinus devices have gradually lost appeal in favor of direct annuloplasties. Although many different technologies have previously been developed, only the *Carillon* (Cardiac Dimensions Inc., Kirkland, WA, USA) remains currently available for clinical use after having obtained CE mark. In patients with implantation success (approx. 68 %), reduction of MR along with functional status improvement has been reported [24].

Other techniques to obtain mitral annulus reduction, such as direct annulus shrinking with different energies [25, 26] or external compression (limited to septo-lateral diameter reduction [27] or complete ventricle restoration), have been proposed. Although very promising, not enough data are available at the moment to judge their clinical value.

## 15.5 Mitral Repair vs Replacement

Mitral repair is widely recognized as superior to replacement in the setting of DMR [28]. In FMR on the other hand, although repair is usually preferred, clear evidence is still lacking [29, 30].

Contrary to what happened in surgery's history, in the next future transcatheter mitral repair will face the competition of replacement. Numerous different mitral prostheses are currently under development and many of them have already reached the clinical phase (Fig. 15.3). However, few compassionate cases have been performed up until now, and the results cannot be judged yet.

Compared to repair, mitral replacement brings the promise to be an easier, more reproducible, more "interventional cardiologist friendly," one-stop-shop procedure; moreover, it should provide a better and more predictable reduction of MR, and it would make of course an ideal landing zone for future valve-in-valve procedures. The prosthesis durability, the presence of paravalvular leaks, the possible need of anticoagulation therapy, and the disruption of physiological hemodynamic function of the mitral valve remain major concerns, however, to be carefully assessed in the future.

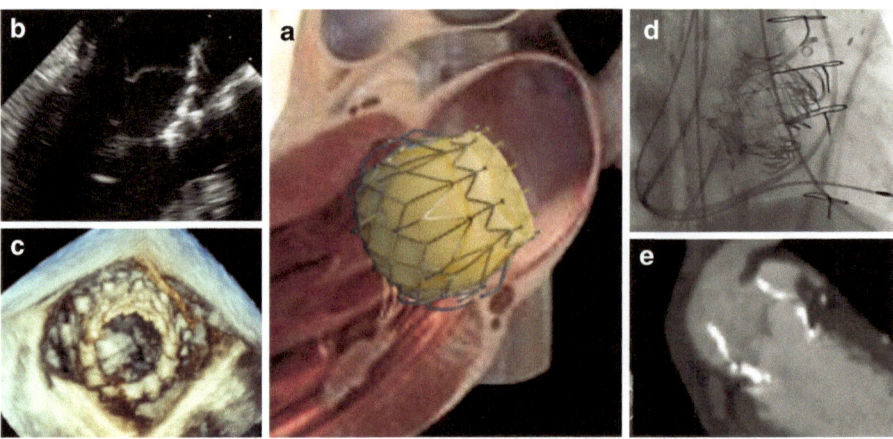

**Fig. 15.3** Mitral valve implantation first-in-man: the CardiAQ Valve. (**a**) Computed simulation of ideal prosthesis position inside the heart; (**b**) 2D echocardiographic appearance after implantation, (**c**) 3D echocardiographic view; (**d**) fluoroscopy view; (**e**) postoperative CT scan assessment confirming good positioning

**Table 15.1** Comparison between theoretical advantages/disadvantages of transcatheter mitral valve repair and replacement

| Repair | Replacement |
| --- | --- |
| More complex | Simpler and more reproducible |
| Needs patient selection/tailored approach | More versatile/same device for every patient |
| Residual MR? | No residual MR? Paravalvular leaks? |
| Durability? | Durability? |
| More natural hemodynamic | Altered hemodynamic |

On the other hand, the repair approach is more difficult and less reproducible; it needs adequate patient selection and multiple devices to reach optimal MR reduction (edge-to-edge/chordal implantation and annuloplasty); it may leave some residual MR and it does not guarantee reliable long-term results yet. However, it would provide a far more natural hemodynamic pattern (Table 15.1) [31, 32].

### Conclusions

The edge-to-edge technique is simple, quick, reproducible, effective, and versatile, allowing the treatment of many different mitral pathologies as no other repair technique (functional MR, Barlow disease, SAM, etc.). The natural evolution of mitral surgery is towards repair rather than replacement and towards minimally invasive/percutaneous approach rather than open surgery. Thanks to its great simplicity and versatility, the edge-to-edge technique perfectly fits both these concepts. Its features will make it one of the leading techniques for the transcatheter treatment of MR in the future, although the addition of other procedures (such as annuloplasty) will be fundamental to reach surgical-like excellent and durable results.

# References

1. Nkomo VT, Gardin JM, Skelton TN, Gottdiener JS, Scott CG, Enriquez-Sarano M. Burden of valvular heart diseases: a population-based study. Lancet. 2006;368:1005–11.
2. Go AS, Mozaffarian D, Roger VL, Benjamin EJ, Berry JD, Blaha MJ, et al. Heart disease and stroke statistics – 2014 update: a report from the American Heart Association. Circulation. 2014;129:e28–292.
3. Mirabel M, Iung B, Baron G, Messika-Zeitoun D, Detaint D, Vanoverschelde JL, et al. What are the characteristics of patients with severe, symptomatic, mitral regurgitation who are denied surgery? Eur Heart J. 2007;28:1358–65.
4. Chiam PT, Ruiz CE. Percutaneous transcatheter mitral valve repair: a classification of the technology. JACC Cardiovasc Interv. 2011;4:1–13.
5. Mauri L, Foster E, Glower DD, Apruzzese P, Massaro JM, Herrmann HC, et al. 4-year results of a randomized controlled trial of percutaneous repair versus surgery for mitral regurgitation. J Am Coll Cardiol. 2013;62:317–28.
6. Vahanian A, Alfieri O, Andreotti F, Antunes MJ, Baron-Esquivias G, Baumgartner H, et al. Guidelines on the management of valvular heart disease (Vers. 2012): The Joint Task Force on the Management of Valvular Heart Disease of the European Society of Cardiology (ESC) and the European Association for Cardio-Thoracic Surgery (EACTS). Eur J Cardiothorac Surg. 2012;42:S1–44.
7. Maisano F, Franzen O, Baldus S, Schafer U, Hausleiter J, Butter C, et al. Percutaneous mitral valve interventions in the real world: early and 1-year results from the Access-EU, a prospective, multicenter, nonrandomized post-approval study of the MitraClip therapy in Europe. J Am Coll Cardiol. 2013;62:1052–61.
8. Nickenig G, Estevez-Loureiro R, Franzen O, Tamburino C, Vanderheyden M, Luscher TF, et al. Percutaneous mitral valve edge-to-edge repair: in-hospital results and 1-year follow-up of 628 patients of the 2011–2012 Pilot European Sentinel Registry. J Am Coll Cardiol. 2014;64:875–84.
9. Seeburger J, Rinaldi M, Nielsen SL, Salizione S, Lange R, Schoenburg M, et al. Off pump transapical implantation of artificial chordae to correct mitral regurgitation (TACT trial) - proof of concept. J Am Coll Cardiol. 2013;63(9):914–9.
10. De Bonis M, Lapenna E, Buzzatti N, Taramasso M, Calabrese MC, Nisi T, et al. Can the edge-to-edge technique provide durable results when used to rescue patients with suboptimal conventional mitral repair? Eur J Cardiothorac Surg. 2013;43:e173–9.
11. Fedak PW, McCarthy PM, Bonow RO. Evolving concepts and technologies in mitral valve repair. Circulation. 2008;117:963–74.
12. Gillinov AM, Tantiwongkosri K, Blackstone EH, Houghtaling PL, Nowicki ER, Sabik III JF, et al. Is prosthetic annuloplasty necessary for durable mitral valve repair? Ann Thorac Surg. 2009;88:76–82.
13. Flameng W, Herijgers P, Bogaerts K. Recurrence of mitral valve regurgitation after mitral valve repair in degenerative valve disease. Circulation. 2003;107:1609–13.
14. De Bonis M, Lapenna E, Maisano F, Barili F, La Canna G, Buzzatti N, et al. Long-term results (</=18 years) of the edge-to-edge mitral valve repair without annuloplasty in degenerative mitral regurgitation: implications for the percutaneous approach. Circulation. 2014;130:S19–24.
15. De Bonis M, Lapenna E, Lorusso R, Buzzati N, Gelsomino S, Taramasso M, et al. Very long-term results (up to 17 years) with the double-orifice mitral valve repair combined with ring annuloplasty for degenerative mitral regurgitation. J Thorac Cardiovasc Surg. 2012;144(5):1019–24.
16. Spoor MT, Geltz A, Bolling SF. Flexible versus nonflexible mitral valve rings for congestive heart failure – differential durability of repair. Circulation. 2006;114:I67–71.
17. Kwon MH, Lee LS, Cevasco M, Couper GS, Shekar PS, Cohn LH, et al. Recurrence of mitral regurgitation after partial versus complete mitral valve ring annuloplasty for functional mitral regurgitation. J Thorac Cardiovasc Surg. 2012;146(3):616–22.

18. Tibayan FA, Rodriguez F, Langer F, Zasio MK, Bailey L, Liang D, et al. Does septal-lateral annular cinching work for chronic ischemic mitral regurgitation? J Thorac Cardiovasc Surg. 2004;127:654–63.

19. Tibayan FA, Rodriguez F, Langer F, Liang D, Daughters GT, Ingels NB, et al. Mitral suture annuloplasty corrects both annular and subvalvular geometry in acute ischemic mitral regurgitation. J Heart Valve Dis. 2004;13:414–20.

20. Bothe W, Kvitting JP, Stephens EH, Swanson JC, Liang DH, Ingels Jr NB, et al. Effects of different annuloplasty ring types on mitral leaflet tenting area during acute myocardial ischemia. J Thorac Cardiovasc Surg. 2011;141:345–53.

21. Maisano F, La Canna G, Latib A, Denti P, Taramasso M, Kuck KH, et al. First-in-man transseptal implantation of a "surgical-like" mitral valve annuloplasty device for functional mitral regurgitation. JACC Cardiovasc Interv. 2014;7(11):1326–8.

22. Siminiak T, Dankowski R, Baszko A, Lee C, Firek L, Kalmucki P, et al. Percutaneous direct mitral annuloplasty using the Mitralign Bident system: description of the method and a case report. Kardiol Pol. 2013;71:1287–92.

23. Tops LF, Van de Veire NR, Schuijf JD, de Roos A, van der Wall EE, Schalij MJ, et al. Noninvasive evaluation of coronary sinus anatomy and its relation to the mitral valve annulus – implications for percutaneous mitral annuloplasty. Circulation. 2007;115:1426–32.

24. Siminiak T, Wu JC, Haude M, Hoppe UC, Sadowski J, Lipiecki J, et al. Treatment of functional mitral regurgitation by percutaneous annuloplasty: results of the TITAN Trial. European J Heart Failure. 2012;14:931–8.

25. Goel R, Witzel T, Dickens D, Takeda PA, Heuser RR. The QuantumCor device for treating mitral regurgitation: an animal study. Catheter Cardiovasc Interv. 2009;74:43–8.

26. Jilaihawi H, Virmani R, Nakagawa H, Ducharme A, Shi YF, Carter-Monroe N, et al. Mitral annular reduction with subablative therapeutic ultrasound: pre-clinical evaluation of the ReCor device. EuroIntervention. 2010;6:54–62.

27. Grossi EA, Patel N, Woo YJ, Goldberg JD, Schwartz CF, Subramanian V, et al. Outcomes of the RESTOR-MV Trial (Randomized Evaluation of a Surgical Treatment for Off-Pump Repair of the Mitral Valve). J Am Coll Cardiol. 2010;56:1984–93.

28. Enriquez-Sarano M, Schaff HV, Orszulak TA, Tajik AJ, Bailey KR, Frye RL. Valve repair improves the outcome of surgery for mitral regurgitation. A multivariate analysis. Circulation. 1995;91:1022–8.

29. Acker MA, Parides MK, Perrault LP, Moskowitz AJ, Gelijns AC, Voisine P, et al. Mitral-valve repair versus replacement for severe ischemic mitral regurgitation. N Engl J Med. 2014;370:23–32.

30. De Bonis M, Ferrara D, Taramasso M, Calabrese MC, Verzini A, Buzzatti N, et al. Mitral replacement or repair for functional mitral regurgitation in dilated and ischemic cardiomyopathy: is it really the same? Ann Thorac Surg. 2012;94:44–51.

31. Pedrizzetti G, La Canna G, Alfieri O, Tonti G. The vortex-an early predictor of cardiovascular outcome? Nat Rev Cardiol. 2014;11(9):545–53.

32. Yacoub MH, Cohn LH. Novel approaches to cardiac valve repair: from structure to function: part I. Circulation. 2004;109:942–50.

# Conclusions

16

## Ottavio Alfieri

The introduction of the edge-to-edge technique was definitely associated with a remarkable positive impact on our clinical practice.

Already in the 1990s our repair rate for degenerative mitral regurgitation was close to 100 %. Furthermore, in contrast with the general experience at that time, similar results for posterior, anterior, bileaflet, and commissural prolapse were obtained.

The edge-to-edge suture was an effective solution when some residual mitral regurgitation was detected immediately after repair and the mechanism responsible for it was not clearly identified. This application considerably contributed to the optimal results of mitral repair in our institution.

Similarly, the systolic anterior movement occasionally complicating mitral repair and producing left ventricular outflow obstruction and residual mitral regurgitation was often effectively corrected with the edge-to-edge suture.

In functional mitral regurgitation the edge-to-edge technique was a valuable addition to annuloplasty in cases with significant tethering and left ventricular remodeling, and valve replacement was only reserved to more advanced situations.

Due to the versatility of the technique, mitral regurgitation could be conveniently corrected through the ventricle during left ventricular restoration procedures, or through the aorta during operations addressing the aortic root, the aortic valve, or the left ventricular outflow tract.

Importantly, the edge-to-edge technique was always only considered an additional tool to be appropriately integrated in the wide armamentarium available to the surgeon to optimally repair the mitral valve.

O. Alfieri, MD, PhD
Cardiac Surgery Unit, IRCCS San Raffaele University Hospital,
Via Olgettina 60, Milan 20132, Italy
e-mail: alfieri.ottavio@hsr.it

© Springer International Publishing Switzerland 2015
O. Alfieri et al. (eds.), *Edge-to-Edge Mitral Repair: From a Surgical to a Percutaneous Approach*, DOI 10.1007/978-3-319-19893-4_16

Currently, only about 15 % of the patients submitted to mitral valve reconstruction in our institution are receiving the edge-to-edge suture as part of the procedure.

Fully aware of the potential problems related to the double-orifice configuration of the mitral valve, we initially applied the new technique with caution.

Moreover, all patients have been carefully evaluated postoperatively over the years (clinically and with echocardiography). Rigorous scientific data have been repeatedly reported by our group in many studies, and are summarized in this book.

Perhaps, from a historical perspective, the most important merit of the edge-to-edge technique was to make percutaneous mitral repair possible.

The simplicity and the effectiveness of this type of mitral valve repair were particularly attractive to innovators exploring methods to correct mitral regurgitation percutaneously via trans-catheter interventions.

The edge-to-edge repair was replicated with the MitraClip system, currently widely used in the clinical practice, and by far the most effective method available today to correct mitral regurgitation percutaneously.

According to the recent European guidelines, the ideal candidate for the clip procedure could be an inoperable or high-risk symptomatic patient with severe mitral regurgitation (organic or functional), fulfilling the echocardiographic criteria of eligibility.

However, the role of the percutaneous clip procedure in the clinical practice is expected to grow in the future for a number of reasons.

Due to the consistent and constant ageing of the population, many more patients suffering from severe mitral regurgitation and too sick to undergo traditional heart surgery will require treatment with relatively safe and well tolerated trans-catheter interventions.

Taking into account the well-documented unfavorable impact of mitral regurgitation on the prognosis, it will be reasonable to consider correction of secondary MR even in patients presenting with only moderate regurgitation and/or without severe symptoms.

The advent of effective catheter-based annuloplasty techniques to be used in combination with the clip procedure is expected to expand the applicability of the MitraClip system and to increase the durability of the percutaneous repair.

In a short time, the percutaneous implantation of a mitral prosthesis will be available as an alternative option for inoperable or high-risk severely symptomatic patients with mitral regurgitation.

It is difficult at this point in time to predict the role of this new procedure in the percutaneous treatment of mitral regurgitation, and to foresee its impact on the MitraClip.

For sure, in the meantime, thousands and thousands of patients will continue to benefit from the percutaneous edge-to-edge repair.